DEPRESSION
Biology, Psychodynamics, and Treatment

DEPRESSION
Biology, Psychodynamics, and Treatment

Edited by

Jonathan O. Cole,

Alan F. Schatzberg,

and

Shervert H. Frazier

McLean Hospital
Belmont, Massachusetts

PLENUM PRESS · NEW YORK AND LONDON

Library of Congress Cataloging in Publication Data

Main entry under title:

Depression.

Chiefly papers presented at a symposium sponsored by McLean Hospital, Belmont, March 28, 1976.

Includes bibliographical references and index.

1. Depression, Mental–Congresses. 2. Mental illness–Physiological aspects–Congresses. 3. Psychopharmacology–Congresses. I. Cole, Jonathan O. II. Schatzberg, Alan F. III. Frazier, Shervert H. [DNLM: 1. Depression–Therapy–Congresses. 2. Depression–Drug therapy–Congresses. WM207 D4145d 1976]

RC537.D4277 616.8'52 77-13161

ISBN 0-306-31062-7

Proceedings of a symposium on depression sponsored by McLean Hospital, Belmont, Massachusetts, March 28, 1976

A Division of Plenum Publishing Corporation
227 West 17th Street, New York, N.Y. 10011

Printed in the United States of America

Contributors

E. JAMES ANTHONY, M.D., Professor of Child Psychiatry, Washington University School of Medicine, St. Louis, Missouri

AARON T. BECK, M.D., Professor of Psychiatry, University of Pennsylvania School of Medicine, Philadelphia, Pennsylvania

DAVID BURNS, M.D., Assistant Professor of Psychiatry, University of Pennsylvania School of Medicine, Philadelphia, Pennsylvania; Fellow of Foundations' Fund for Research in Psychiatry

JANE F. CAHILL, R.N., Nurse, Neuropsychopharmacology Laboratory, Massachusetts Mental Health Center, Boston, Massachusetts

PIETRO CASTELNUOVO-TEDESCO, M.D., James G. Blakemore Professor of Psychiatry, Vanderbilt University School of Medicine, Nashville, Tennessee

JONATHAN O. COLE, M.D., Director, Psychopharmacology, McLean Hospital, Belmont, Massachusetts

SHERVERT H. FRAZIER, M.D., Psychiatrist in Chief, McLean Hospital, Belmont, Massachusetts; Professor of Psychiatry, Harvard Medical School, Boston, Massachusetts

DANIEL X. FREEDMAN, M.D., Louis Block Professor of Biological Sciences, Chairman, Department of Psychiatry, University of Chicago, Chicago, Illinois

ROBERT W. GIBSON, M.D., Medical Director, Sheppard and Enoch Pratt Hospital, Towson, Maryland

FREDERICK K. GOODWIN, M.D., Chief, Clinical Psychobiology Branch, National Institute of Mental Health, Bethesda, Maryland

JON E. GUDEMAN, M.D., Associate Professor of Psychiatry, Harvard Medical School, Boston, Massachusetts

LEO E. HOLLISTER, M.D., Professor of Medicine and Psychiatry, Stanford University School of Medicine, Palo Alto, California

PHILLIP L. ISENBERG, M.D., Assistant Professor of Psychiatry, Harvard Medical School, Boston, Massachusetts

KENNETH K. KIDD, M.D., Associate Professor of Human Genetics, Yale University School of Medicine, New Haven, Connecticut

GERALD L. KLERMAN, M.D., Director, Stanley Cobb Psychiatric Research Laboratories, Psychiatry Service, Massachusetts General Hospital; Professor of Psychiatry, Harvard Medical School, Boston, Massachusetts

NATHAN S. KLINE, M.D., Director, Rockland Research Institute, Orangeburg, New York

RICHARD A. LABRIE, Ph.D., Statistical Consultant, Neuropsychopharmacology Laboratory, Massachusetts Mental Health Center, Boston, Massachusetts

PAUL J. ORSULAK, Ph.D., Biochemist, Neuropsychopharmacology Laboratory, Massachusetts Mental Health Center, Boston, Massachusetts

WILLIAM Z. POTTER, M.D., Clinical Associate, Clinical Psychobiology Branch, National Institute of Mental Health, Bethesda, Maryland

WILLIAM A. ROHDE, M.D., Instructor in Psychiatry, Harvard Medical School, Boston, Massachusetts

ALAN F. SCHATZBERG, M.D., Co-Director, Affective Disease Program, McLean Hospital, Belmont, Massachusetts; Instructor in Psychiatry, Harvard Medical School, Boston, Massachusetts

JOSEPH J. SCHILDKRAUT, M.D., Professor of Psychiatry, Harvard Medical School, Boston, Massachusetts; Director, Neuropsychopharmacology Laboratory, Massachusetts Mental Health Center, Boston, Massachusetts

MYRNA M. WEISSMAN, Ph.D., Assistant Professor of Psychiatry (Epidemiology), Yale University School of Medicine, New Haven, Connecticut

Preface

I have of late—but wherefore I know not—lost all my mirth, foregone all custom of exercises, and indeed it goes so heavily with my disposition that this goodly frame, the earth, seems to me a sterile promontory. . . .

Hamlet, in *Hamlet*, Act II, Sc. 2.

The numbers may have been fewer in Shakespeare's time, but the symptoms were the same. Now, each year, millions instead of thousands of people suffer from a clinical depression severe enough for them to seek help from medical and mental health practitioners. Depression is the most common of all psychiatric disorders and affects people of all ages—from childhood to senescence. Since it represents a major medical, public health, and social problem for our culture, it is vitally important that physicians and mental health professionals of all disciplines have a current and thorough understanding of various aspects of the illness—its etiologies, biology, dynamics, course, treatment, and, in some cases, its long-term management.

Depression has long been known to Western civilization with early references to it dating back to Homeric writings. In subsequent times, works of art have often portrayed individuals suffering from depression, and medical tomes have proposed a host of therapies, most of which are antiquated. Over time, however, our knowledge has steadily grown. Psychoanalytic theory and observations have added to our understanding of the depressed patient's psychology and dynamics. More recently, breakthroughs in neurotransmitter research are opening ways to a more basic understanding of the nosology and treatment of the illness. There is now some evidence that manic-depressive illness has a genetic basis. In addition, we are now beginning to see that patients' depressions may be classified on the basis of catecholamine metabolite excretion and that responsiveness to one or another tricyclic medication may ultimately be predictable. Treatment and prevention efficacies have been increased recently with the advent of tricyclic serum levels and the expanded use of lithium. Clearly, with our horizons broadening rapidly, it is essential that we all be familiar with the most current work on the biologic bases, psychodynamic theory and treatments, and psychopharmacological approaches. This need and the ubiquity of the illness led us to hold a McLean Hospital symposium on depression in Boston on March 28, 1976, in cooperation with the Massachusetts Psychiatric Society and the Massachusetts Academy of Family Physicians. The symposium presented recent work by leading investigators on the biology and treatment (both psychopharmacologic and psychotherapeutic) of depression. Many of the chapters in this book are based on papers presented at the conference. Also, several chapters have been added to provide the reader with a comprehensive and basic view of depressive disorders beyond that which is possible in a one-day conference. Material, including recent research, is presented with an eye toward supporting clinicians' efforts at treating depressed patients, in the hope that patients of today and tomorrow can be helped to suffer less than they or others had in the past.

A book such as this could not be completed without the help of many whose names do not appear as principals in the text. In particular, we wish to thank Mrs. Evelyn M. Stone, whose editing, dedication, and hard effort are largely responsible for this volume. Too, Mrs. Sophie Weinfield and Ms. Jean Sanford aided greatly in proofreading and preparing the manuscript. Last, our appreciation is extended to Geigy Pharmaceuticals, who generously supported the Depression Symposium.

Jonathan O. Cole
Alan F. Schatzberg
Shervert H. Frazier

Belmont, Massachusetts

Contents

DEPRESSION
Biology, Psychodynamics, and Treatment

Introduction

DANIEL X. FREEDMAN

In writing this introduction, I feel relieved of the task—not seriously assigned to me, thankfully—of summarizing what depression *really* is. As with any major disorder with multiple determinants, it is convenient to "lump" phenomena into a simple, comprehensible psychological or psychobiological grouping. Thus, we can see a nonnegotiable symptom complex in which the dynamics of loss, hopelessness, ambivalence, and introverted anger play their role, based on historically determined vulnerabilities in the regulation of self-esteem, "adgression," and object relations. We can view the lack of coping, the redundancy of thought processes, the attentional fixation—the general lack of behavioral output with its vegetative and psychological concomitants—as an organismic conservation–withdrawal response. We can see these responses as *triggered* through stress, as the individual has been "prepared" for it through developmental vicissitudes or biological vulnerabilities, and *sustained* perhaps by a different weighting of somatic and psychological factors. The fixation of depressive behavior, its intransigence—this aspect represents a possibly different constellation of issues and psychobiological consequences from issues of vulnerability and resistance to recurrence.

But if we shift our scope to a higher-power focus, these generalities dissolve as the "lumpers" give way to the "splitters," searching out subgroups based on symptomatic, familial, and genetic characteristics, on biological measures or therapeutic response, or on outcome. Such special focus is necessary to implement specific inquiry to account for similarities and differences along these dimensions. And this has characterized the past decade.

DANIEL X. FREEDMAN • Department of Psychiatry, University of Chicago, Chicago, Illinois.

Without ignoring the absolutely astonishing rate of new and clearly established knowledge, we still must regard our efforts in some perspective. Long ago, Walter von Bayer remarked on depression as "the empty space between the uncomprehended psychological and the unexplained somatic."[1] We fill that gap with our various diagnostic, psychodynamic, psychobiologic, and epidemiologic efforts—and even more with our speculations. Yet it is impossible in modern scientific medicine to be intolerant of or impatient with complexity and ambiguity. We are required—by our knowledge of the way things are—to keep varied perspectives simultaneously in mind, and varied tasks as well. The task of understanding the interacting sequences and phases of somatopsychic events with respect to etiology, course, and outcome should require no sermon in its support. The task of diagnosing the condition, the study of the person with a condition, and the understanding of his specific situation with its (and his) resources and stresses may lead to quite specific selections of therapeutic approaches—and the difficulty is that these will not always be directly guided by what research is learning of the multiple mechanisms for the different phases of depressive disorders.

The informed pragmatism of clinical medicine, in brief, pertains to the treatment of depression as well as of any other major dysfunction. In the choice of therapy the physician always keeps in mind the person who is a patient—his reactivity to and use of interventions—as well as the disorder the patient endures. The polarized antinomy of the robot actions of the mechanistic psychiatrist who only dispenses a cocktail to a computerized diagnosis rather than to a person versus the tender solipsism of the "spiritualist" therapist is an obvious exaggeration and distortion of the knowledge and purpose with which we approach the patient and prescribe therapy. It is hard to find a disease process which is treatable solely by drug regardless of personality traits, allergies, idiosyncratic traits, and the "behavings" of the patient. (Witness the current furor of attention on "patient compliance" in chronic disease—and the rush of *both* behavioral scientists *and* an odd lot of "behavior controllers" to aid the medical clinics.) Nor, given our scientific knowledge, is there any support for a "spiritualist" view that there is no psychobiological organization that can play a role in impairing the capacity of the individual to implement his intentions.

In an era of effective medications that can help a significant number of depressed patients, it is of special importance to reach the person who is the patient and to see to what extent he can be mobilized to be a participant in his destiny. In an era when we are challenged to become better phenomenologists, with an improved focus on differential diagnosis (in which we know, for example, of the "many faces of mania"), the issue for the therapist is to determine the practical sequence of interventions useful for a particular patient. Patients have histories, personalities, skills, defects, and biases. The symptoms are often egosyntonic and wish fulfilling, maintained by rewards difficult to grasp without searching behavioral and psychodynamic analysis. The remitted depressive may have to learn about his habits of thought and modes of relating to himself and others. All this is a part of the total assessment by an informed psychiatrist—it is in his mind as he approaches the particular case. In the presence of pyrexia, right lower quadrant abdominal pain, and lymphocytosis, the physician does not probe the hypothalamus although he rightly knows temperature regulation is mediated there. Rather, he selects what is proximal, possible, and practical in whatever phase of intervention he engages the patient. If he does not engage in combined pharmacotherapy and psychotherapy it is *not* because he does not know how, but rather that he deliberately chooses not to do so. The physician surely borrows the wisdom of Ecclesiastes in determining the appropriate time for particular reapings and sowings.

Thus, if he is informed, the psychiatrist will not withhold truly adequate dosage of pharmacotherapy nor overlook the decision about possible maintenance treatment for the remitted patient. If he is at all experienced with the range of real clinical phenomena, he could not fail to notice that for some of the severe depressions psychotherapy—especially in remitted depression—can bring an edge of advantage to the patient. Building on the prior therapeutic relationship, the patient may learn to cope differently, to exert some control over his behavior. If he is a cycling patient he may be able to exert some action as his inspection of his own swings provides both recognition of and response to previously ignored early warning signs. It is no insult to the psychotherapist or to the patient's autonomy if he learns this while on a regimen of lithium—and, in brief, collaborates in his own self-regulation. In a secondary—postviral—depression, it is clearly relevant to help the patient learn not to exhaust himself in useless battle against the viral-induced limitation of energy span. In primary depression, it is not trivial to overlook the capacity of many patients to enhance a break by "letting go" and, conversely, to gain some mastery and perspective over these impulses and traits. One manic patient, 28 years old, appearing to be resistant to lithium was, on closer investigation, a remarkably canny chemist. He loaded himself with popcorn, salt, and water, diuresing lithium in order to be free of whatever psychomotor slowing it is that lithium provides. Lacking this chemically induced "pause" between impulse and action, he not only was free to act up but was soon in the grips of being unable *not* to act up. After dealing with some of his angers toward his family and his perceptions of where the task of control truly lay (of who was trying to control whom), he became a steadily maintained lithium "success."

These considerations forbid any glib, automated approach to the major depressions. If we accept what Klerman has emphasized in Chapter 13—that the majority of depressions do lie outside the limited scope of prototypical unipolar or bipolar depression (for which highly rigid criteria are necessary if useful research is to proceed)—we should pause briefly to understand the rationale for any kind of intervention in depression. In the prepharmacotherapy era, marked by an irrational rejection of ECT (which wounded the vanity of the newly trained psychotherapist even more than that of his analytic teachers), it was possible for physician and patient to maintain a communal watch over agonizing psychic pain for six, nine, or twelve months and to witness the resolution of the severely impairing episode—whether it had run its course or responded to the patience and persistence of the treating staff. Recently, a former student of that era chastised me for now advising medication. He was reacting in part to the invitation to blithe mechanization of the status of persons in trouble. That it is neither more scientific nor more humane to steer the person into becoming either a pill repository or a suffering communicant and spiritual brother is clear. Yet—aside from the grim fact that 5–15% of major depressions did *not* improve (and the impact of modern somatotherapy on these is yet unclear)—a majority did eventually improve without specific therapy.

Thus, it is worth considering the sanction for the psychiatric physician who is disposed to treat the range of depressions with available somatic therapies. The enduring sanction, of course, applies to all medicine and psychological intervention: we deal with authentic suffering. In the great majority of cases the individual who is suffering is not content with his state and his colleagues certainly are not. But we also deal with more than suffering. We deal with people who are more than limited—with individuals who, because of their limitation and suffering, are exploitable by their families, by their competitive colleagues, and by their friends (and unsolicited contemporary "advocates" as well!). This is true whether we deal with a manic or a suicidal patient. The patient is at a social disadvantage and his interactions and transactions are at risk as the very complicated and ambivalent attitudes of those about him interact with his own (often exploitative) modes of relating to them. So I think the sanction we borrow is the classic medical one: to be humanistic in the face of vulnerability and suffering and if we have useful scientific knowledge to apply it with care.

Finally, if neither science nor humanism is served by ideologies that distract us from comprehending complexity, then we should stop being distracted by loose pejorative chitchat about the "medical model"; such parlance is too frequently, covertly used to caricature a "medicines model." "Behavior control," violations of autonomy, of bodily and personal integrity—these are *not* the aim and do not comprise the actual complexity of practices in medicine. Rather, we must observe the physician's true orientation and function.

The true task of medicine is to enhance optimal self-regulation—whether of dysfunctional organs or dysfunctional perception and impairment in implementing personal intent. The medical task, in brief, is to help the organism to establish a viable equilibrium. In so doing we do not have "behavioral control" in mind, nor is a "Clockwork Orange" within our grasp—in fact, not even a clockwork lemon! That respect for self-regulation can be breached by irreverent moonlike persuasions and "Gaslight" perversions of trust or unethical doping of consciousness is clear. But therapeutic measures—including ECT—are a part of a *sequence* and the aim is for the patient to achieve maximal autonomy of function, an aim in fact more frequently achieved than not! The medical model utilizes medicines as part of a total treatment procedure, not as ends in themselves.

So, in 1977 there is no question that with our store of therapeutic skills, medicines, and diagnosis (with careful attention to phenomenology and history taking), there has been a distinct change in our ability to help. This change should be striking to those of us who have long trained a variety of residents (and probably miseducated them over a period of time!). It is striking when one proceeds to a state hospital to rediagnose and treat many so-called schizophrenics whose irritability, diurnal variation in mood, sleep, and vegetative function, and paranoid and schizophreniform symptoms are evident. Such patients, in fact, are found to be reacting, according to their repetoire of available behaviors, to something like a disease process we call depression! E. H. Uhlenhuth in our hospital has found that with this kind of attention to detail one can select outpatients for tests with new antianxiety agents. Those who are jittery, irritable, and denying depression but who on inquiry show vegetative signs of depression can be sorted out. The gain, interestingly, is that it is thus possible to help the truly anxious patient by not masking the effectiveness of an antianxiety drug with tests of a heterogeneous group. It is equally clear that antianxiety drugs, often without clear warrant, have been charged with generating suicidal thoughts when they were in fact mistakenly prescribed in undiagnosed depression.

Similarly, we can see a new interest and focus in the cycloid, atypical, reactive, or schizophreniform dysfunctions.[2,3] These had been noted by Kraepelin,[4] and in 1933 New England's Kasanin,[5] followed later by Stanley Cobb,[6] focused on "schizoaffective" psychoses. However these issues are sorted out, investigation will be of practical use in the search for more specific therapeutic approaches in psychiatry. Recently, the University of Pittsburgh group has identified therapeutically resistant populations of severe depressions, persons showing simultaneously manic and depressive features or rapidly cycling; they are found on inquiry to also be substance abusers (especially of alcohol).[7] These groups may show 40% or 50% failure on therapeutic regimens normally effective for depression.

So this keener differentiation and alertness to a variety of factors may enhance whatever therapeutic regimen is selected and certainly brings a vastly different picture to the treatment of depression in American psychiatry from one that could have been summoned a decade ago. Nor should we neglect the election of ECT as a treatment or research into not only its mode of action but the psychological variables and adaptations entailed in recovery induced by ECT. The data show fewer deaths in ECT than in drug treatment—until one parcels out adequately dosed patients.[8] The often remarked anxiety and dysphoria seen after four or five treatments and the psychodynamic motives in different patterns of utilization of memory loss may evoke research interest. One severely depressed patient, for example, after six ECT treatments lost his general denial of his wife's death and remembered the pain of loss and its details, eventually working it through a process of mourning.

Another major open question to be explored is the role of physical and psychological developmental status and the depressive symptomatic state. Exactly what kind of development of personality and ego functions is necessary for the prototypical, obsessional symptoms and rigidities of the involutional melancholic? David Hawkins has noted to me the fact that adolescents with severe mood disorders sleep a lot instead of showing early-morning wakings and the like. These are not insignificant questions, in terms of both the psychobiology of depression and the interaction of ego structure and personality traits with the disorder. Do young Class Four patients have a more "consolidated" personality at a younger age than that achieved by the introspective college student? If so, when depressed, do they manifest classic depressive symptoms earlier than our protean late adolescents? Many clinicians today see depressed adolescents in adolescent turmoil in which the focus of self-attention is on mood rather than on regulated action. When with advancing age does a more classic depressive syndrome appear in these cases? In brief, are we dealing with similar processes in classic and adolescent depression which are differently manifested because of the developmental status and intrapsychic organization of these patients? Is their psychobiological status in depression different or similar? Why do we not have as good data on infant and childhood at risk measures of psychobiological function for manic-depression as are available for genetic schizophrenia? (See Chapter 10 by Anthony.)

In any event, for depressive disorders of adulthood it is clear that many, if not all, therapies rely on some sort of mobilization of behavioral output. The tricyclics seem to affect motoric activity—to have something to do with the mobilization of behavior. While we need to know more of their effects in normals, the tricyclics do not seem primarily to affect mood or the varied existential postures of hope. (The manipulation of moods seems far more the province of the depressed alcoholic and heroin addict—or of adolescents who play upon mood with an array of romances and a wide variety of street drugs which affect momentary state.) Perhaps it is useful to look at the psychology of depression, the pacing, agitation, and self-castigation, as incomplete restitutive attempts to mobilize output.

The effect of therapy such as Beck and Burns report in Chapter 12 is similar (the mock courtroom scene to which the patient seems aroused, reacting with an initial interest and detached amusement to his mobilization). Twenty years ago we thought of how to get patients angry and to begin to express themselves. In brief, it is possible that in depression we are dealing psychologically and psychobiologically with a kind of massive inhibition, on the one hand, and with self-initiated attempts to move out of that inhibition, which we therapeutically attempt to influence. There is indeed a psychobiological dimension related to mobilization and implementation of motoric behavior which has long been evident in studies of the retardation, akinesia, and inertia in Parkinsonism. The "start" mechanism, even when intended, is difficult to activate, and Arnold Mandell and colleagues noted that with tricyclic therapy of Parkinsonians this was the first symptom to respond.[9] That is mobilization toward output may be a dopamine-mediated function which is enhanced by the overlooked dopamine-sparing effects of tricyclics has been commented on elsewhere by Halaris and myself.[10] Inflexibility in the biological responses of depression was noted in the lack of hormonal responsivity to insulin and lack of the expected diurnal characteristics of cortisone secretion rate by Sachar's group. Psychologically the grim and intensive focus on self, the thought disorder which Beck and Burns later explicate, and the lack of differentiated coping behaviors raise the question of whether we are dealing primarily with a mood disorder or with a disorder of the control of rate by which different biopsychological subsystems (perhaps limbic–midbrain systems) become rigidly locked into place and resistant to ordinary input. Thus more than mood is to be investigated and it should be noted that there is a mobilizing but noneuphoric effect of cocaine in severe depression. This cautions us from facilely conceiving of euphoria and depression as direct polar opposites; at least in terms of investigating their biobehavioral initiating or mediating infrastructures, this may not be a fully adequate notion.

As we step back and take some perspective of how we now comprehend the role of biogenic amines in affective disorders, such reflections may also be relevant. At some juncture we must ask ultimately what the amines mean. With what other ongoing neural organization do changes in aminergic neural systems interact? While my own research has long been directed to "aminology," I believe, both for basic biobehavioral studies and for the application of these to the neurobiology of clinical disorder, some perspective on more than "juices"—chemicals—will be required. Simplistically, we deal with both "juices" and "wires," and it is well to remember that the brain is "built" to behave; its ongoing behavioral disposition and activity is keyed to the influence of the next signal or input. If we simply study rates of behavioral output, we know that animals or man already responding at a low rate will increase output in the presence of amphetamines, or, if they are working at a high rate, the drug will then decrease it. The sedation threshold of Shagass[11] and Perez–Reyes[12] clearly indicates a different prior state, one readily shifted by barbiturates in the case of psychotic depression as compared to milder depressive states. All this is to the point that we must avoid thinking simplistically of the link of amines to neurobehavioral systems. Dr. Barbara Jones[13] at the University of Chicago recently demonstrated that a lesion depleting the cortex of all of its norepinephrine does not affect the regulation of sleep, sleep phases, or activation. On the other hand, if the amines are partially depleted, they do have some influence on the regulation of the basic biological processes governing sleep stages, activation, and arousal.

In brief, the presence of the amine may have something to do with the ongoing state of the neuron and its interregulations, but the "juices" need not be conceived of as "forcing" behavioral states upon organized neuronal systems. So, accepting the notion that the ongoing business of the brain is to adapt and implement behavior, it is difficult to think of it as specifically controlled in its fundamental behavioral adaptations by "juices." While such a view may be misleading, the role of amines on the operations of different neural nets can be conceived of as modulating ongoing rates of these different brain systems—differentially affecting them but according to their prior organization and state. Drugs affecting amines may shift the response in certain neural systems, thereby enhancing or diminishing the activity of others—in brief, drugs permit the establishment of a new equilibrium. But the pathways that create fundamental disequilibria postulated in disease may be many. It thus may really be naive to think of a "one juice–one disease" correlation. As an example, there are startling data of Shopsin, Friedman, and Gershon[14] indicating that inhibition of norepinephrine synthesis does not impair the effectiveness of tricyclic antidepressants or MAO inhibitors in treating severe depression (whereas a slight decrease in serotonin synthesis drastically does); this clearly indicates why we should be cautious of any simplistic catecholamine model of depression or of the therapeutic mode of action of drugs in depression. Perhaps we should remember that amphetamine was once a model antidepressant and currently is a model for schizophrenia; reserpine was an antischizophrenic and became a model depression; postencephalitic Parkinsonism was an organic model for schizophrenia and current dopaminergic blockade therapy would have us postulate that Parkinsonism would be antithetical to schizophrenia. While there are chemicals that may produce a "model psychosis" in man, I know of none (including reserpine) that directly *and* reliably produce a "model depression." The first law of psychopharmacology should be, to preach my favorite sermon, "prior state," and this factor may well explain the many variabilities observed with amine precursors and enzyme inhibitors in normal and diseased man. Apart from cautioning us not to deduce the organization of the nervous system simplistically, the status of current revolutions in neurobiology forces us to anticipate change. For example, the discovery of a drug that might act rapidly to reverse depression without primary action on monoamines would strike a serious blow to current metapharmacology.

Nevertheless, by tracing the effects of drugs on central aminergic systems, we have for the first time gotten a grip not only on the multiple mechanisms by which drugs change brain chemistry and behavior but on relevant measures of brain biochemistry to be studied in man. We can always hope that the effect of a drug will lead us to a causal effect of the initial disequilibrium, but we cannot rely on that; digitalis affects the force and contraction of the heart but does not lead us to the cause of cardiac decompensation. If the brain can be variably influenced to find a more adaptive new equilibrium with therapy, this should be sufficient in its own right. Thus, even though we have no guarantee of their basic theoretical significance, we must look with great hope for the practical consequences of the studies by the NIMH group and Schildkraut (detailed in Chapters 2 and 3) on the amine status of depressed persons prior to treatment and on possible predictors for differential therapeutic response. What we will someday have to remember is that, of the billions of brain cells, the 6000 or so neurons that synthesize amines project in discrete systems to a very wide variety of neural aggregates; they are but a component of the working brain. The neurobiological thrust of the early 1950s will have to be reapproached with studies of the neurobehavioral consequences of limbic systems as well as the newly characterized specific neocortical receptor systems to which many of the amine cells project. In summary, while we still do not fully know the psychobiology of depression but rather have some grasp of components of it and while we cannot make a logically coherent story out of biobehavioral substrate of this clinical disorder, there does seem to be sound evidence of the lack of adaptive regulation and lack of differentiation of functions in depression, and from such evidence there may be some practical spin-off.

To be futuristic, it is possible that general hospital psychiatry will regularly utilize estimates of catecholamine status to select one or another drug and to utilize, as well, radioimmune assay of drug levels to monitor adequate dosage regimens. We should soon systematically measure lithium red blood cell concentration, which promises to more faithfully guide lithium therapy and dosage than plasma levels in "resistant" cases. The dexamethasone suppression test, currently investigated by Bernard Carroll[15] and others, may become a useful diagnostic tool, since it appears that the expected diurnal suppression induced by the drug does not occur in severe depression. Studies of sleep dysfunction (of shortened REM latency) may also be usefully diagnostic and, as the Pittsburgh group suggests, REM density may be one measure for identifying medical versus the primary psychiatrically relevant depressions.

But we finally must turn to the issue of adequate funds and manpower. It is an issue about which we should be situationally depressed but hopefully mobilized in a therapeutically affective way. The striking fact is that we have available a cadre of clinically trained psychiatrists capable of biochemical, neurobiological, and psychodiagnostic and epidemiologic research. The concentrated neglect in the past ten years in our capacity not only to undertake research but to generate the knowledgeable manpower for it ironically occurs exactly at a time when the state of the art of the sciences in psychiatry provides the strongest warrant for research and research manpower investment in the entire history of psychiatry. I do not regret the studied neglect when I think of seasoned researchers; but I am concerned for the patients whose suffering is still our charge and for whom we lack the specificity and potency of treatment that we and they would desire—even though we are in far better shape than a quarter of a century ago.

I especially regret the message we are giving to young people whom we are quickly getting to the point of being unable to train. The leads and findings we are discussing in this book were in fact put into motion twenty and some many more years ago. We cannot count on that momentum either to pursue the leads now in hand or to develop those that the logic of science indicates can readily be generated. Nationally we spend about twenty dollars for research for each ill patient under care for mental illness—perhaps three to four million persons at any one time for whom new and effective knowledge should be welcome. For comparison we may spend perhaps ninety dollars per patient under care for heart disease and two hundred dollars for cancer. It is not really self-serving to advocate mobilizing ourselves to capitalize on the chances for new knowledge and for the development and articulation of findings that are really at hand. So we have an unexpected additional professional task: in concert with the vast range of those who care, to alert professional self-respect, public concern—and hope. For that hope, this book provides a sound testament.

REFERENCES

1. Bayer W von: Zur Psychopathologie der endogenen Psychosen. *Nervenarzt 24:*316, 1953.
2. Tsuang M, Dempsey M, Rauscher F: A study of "atypical schizophrenia." *Arch. Gen. Psychiatry 33:*1157–1160, 1976.
3. Procci WR: Schizo-affective psychosis: Fact or fiction? *Arch. Gen. Psychiatry 33:*1167–1178, 1976.
4. Kraepelin E: *Clinical Psychiatry.* (Translated from Seventh German Edition by Diefendorf AR.) New York, Macmillan, 1923.
5. Kasanin J: The acute schizoaffective psychoses. *Am. J. Psychiatry 13:*97–126, 1933.
6. Cobb S: *Borderline of Psychiatry.* Cambridge, Harvard University Press, 1943.
7. Himmelhoch JM, Mulla D, Neil JF, Detre TP, Kupfer DJ: Incidence and significance of mixed affective states in a bipolar population. *Arch. Gen. Psychiatry 33:*1062–1066, 1976.
8. Avery D, Winokur G: Mortality in depressed patients treated with electroconvulsive therapy and antidepressants. *Arch. Gen. Psychiatry 33:*1029–1037, 1976.
9. Mandell AJ, Markham C, Fowler W: Parkinson's syndrome, depression and imipramine. *Calif. Med. 95:*12–14.
10. Halaris A, Freedman DX: Psychotropic drugs and dopamine uptake inhibition. In: Freedman DX (ed) *Biology of the Major Psychosis: A Comparative Analysis,* Research Publications Vol. 54, pp. 247–258. New York, Raven Press, 1975.
11. Shagass, CS, Naiman J, Mihalik J: An objective test which differentiates between neurotic and psychotic depression. *Arch. Neurol. Psychiatry 75:*461, 1956.
12. Perez-Reyes M: Differences in sedative susceptibility between types of depression: Clinical and neurophysiological significance. *Arch. Gen. Psychiatry 19:*64–71, 1968.
13. Jones BE, Harper ST, Halaris AE: Effects of locus coeruleus lesions upon cerebral monoamine content, sleep-wakefulness states and the response to amphetamine in the cat. *Brain Res. 124:*473–496, 1977.
14. Shopsin B, Friedman E, Gershon S: Parachlorophenylalanine reversal of tranylcypromine in depressed patients. *Arch. Gen. Psychiatry 33:*811–819, 1976.
15. Carroll BJ, Curtis GC, Mendels J: Neuroendocrine regulation in depression. II. Discrimination of depressed from nondepressed patients. *Arch. Gen. Psychiatry 33:*1051–1058, 1976.

1

Classification of Depressive Disorders

ALAN F. SCHATZBERG

The recent advent of effective psychopharmacologic treatments for subtypes of depressive disorders has converted the classification of the depressions from an academic exercise to a pragmatic necessity for good patient care. Advances in the biology and treatment of depression (exemplified clearly in the remainder of this book) have enabled workers and practitioners to begin to solve those unanswered questions which had previously limited treatment efficacy. In fact, so amorphous was the state of knowledge of etiology and treatment that some workers such as the British psychiatrist Mapother argued in 1926 that classification was of little practical value:

> It will be generally agreed that subdivision in virtue of details of the known (for example, of past course and present symptoms) serves little purpose unless the types discriminated are correlated with the differences in the unknown—for example in causation, prognosis, or treatment.[1]

However, 50 years have passed, and recent advances in biology and treatment have dictated that the practitioner of today must have a working knowledge of current diagnosis and classification if he is to treat the depressed patient effectively. In addition, investigators believed that efficient and precise classification fosters further research on etiology.[2,3] Indeed, as will be demonstrated in this chapter, many of the more recent classification systems have been proposed by researchers. In short, classification of depressive disorders can no longer be viewed as an intellectual game but rather as a cornerstone of comprehensive understanding and treatment.

ALAN F. SCHATZBERG • McLean Hospital, Belmont, Massachusetts, and Department of Psychiatry, Harvard Medical School, Boston, Massachusetts.

Unfortunately, however, the classification of depressive disorders continues to be an area of intellectual debate as it has been for the past 70 years. Classification is a constantly evolving process, many systems having been proposed over the years, each with its strengths and weaknesses. Globally, classifications have been divided into two approaches: dimensional and categorical. In the dimensional approach, depression is viewed primarily as a spectrum of a unitary disorder; in the more popular categorical one, it may be grouped under one disorder but more commonly is divided into two (binary) or more (pluralistic) subgroups. Further, dimensional and categorical approaches contain many individual systems, and differences often exist between systems. Part of the variance reflects the fact that systems have been generated by researchers and clinicians working at different times, in different locales, and with singular areas of interest. Also, an individual system has often tended to reflect the psychiatric thinking and knowledge of the time as well as the available research technology. Thus, the works of Kraepelin (1904, 1921)[4,5] and Lewis (1934)[6]—based on extensive case studies—are quite different from those of Hamilton and White (1959)[7]—which utilized factor analysis and computers. Further, recent workers have employed data on clinical outcome, genetics, and biology in developing classification systems—a state of affairs quite different from the pioneer days of Kraepelin, Lewis, Mapother, and others.

Although systems have become increasingly refined, differences still exist as to specific criteria for diagnosis (e.g., symptoms, course, biology, genetics, etc.), the definition of terms/variables, the relationship or clustering of variables, and the clinical significance of subdivisions, let alone which is the best approach or system. Taken as a whole, the literature on classification is often confusing. However, as Kendell[8] has noted, clear agreement has begun to emerge on several major issues: the definition and existence of an endogenous syndrome; the differentiation between unipolar and bipolar depressions; and the view that involutional melancholia is a needless term since it reflects a unipolar, agitated depression which may occur at ages other than the climacterium. Although this last point has achieved considerable popularity, in my view it is still open to some question.

In this chapter, aspects of the classification debate are reviewed and attempts are made to dissect and trace some of the major issues, confusions, and controversies. Several systems, including the current DSMII classification, are reviewed in terms of their strengths and weaknesses and some recent classifications are presented with an eye toward anticipating where further work may lead us. Since a comprehensive review of the literature is beyond the scope of this chapter, I have limited my review to the more important and representative works and have emphasized the pragmatic aspects of classification. The reader is referred elsewhere for further discussions on classifications.[8–14]

ENDOGENOUS VS. NONENDOGENOUS

For many years, a major area of debate has centered around the endogenous and nonendogenous states, particularly their relationship and their criteria for definition. Some have maintained that endogenous and nonendogenous states represent poles of a spectrum[13,15]; others, that all depressions may be classified into endogenous or nonendogenous states (i.e., an all-inclusive dichotomy)[2]; and others, that endogenous states represent "classic depressions" while their nonendogenous counterparts consist of a group of assorted, often neurotic, disorders[12,16]; and a last group, that endogenous and nonendogenous groups are two subtypes of a larger system.[17]

The endogenous/nonendogenous distinction began with Kraepelin, who separated the two groups primarily on the basis of precipitation, a premise which some later workers have questioned. Subsequently, investigators have proposed a host of other differentiating criteria, including symptom clusters, reactivity of symptoms, premorbid personality, guilt/blame, family history, etc. However, there has been no clear agreement about the significance and definition of all these variables or dimensions and how they are related. Workers have often defined the same term (e.g., psychosis) in rather different ways and have used different terms (which had traditionally often referred to rather discrete dimensions) to describe a single phenomenon. The latter is exemplified by the use of the terms *autonomous* and *psychotic* to describe endogenous states and the use of the terms *reactive, psychogenic, exogenous,* and *neurotic* for their nonendogenous counterparts. The end result has been rather complex and often confusing.

Some agreement, however, has emerged as to the existence and symptom criteria for an endogenous syndrome.[8] Such unanimity is lacking in regard to its nonendogenous counterpart; some workers have debated against its existence as a depressive state while others have proposed several different subtypes. Early investigators tended to define the symptoms of a nonendogenous state negatively, i.e., nonendogenous symptoms did not exist but merely meant that endogenous ones were absent. Later works described positive criteria for several types of nonendogenous depressions, but some of these states may appear to be more neurotic or characterologic than depressive. The inability to define a clear-cut nonendogenous state has undoubtedly weakened the argument that a clear dichotomy exists.

The remainder of this section attempts to highlight the history of this major debate and to review and trace some of the issues, controversies, and confusion. The discussion is divided into early and later work since investigative tools and manners of presentation and validation have varied greatly over the years.

Early Writings

In his pioneer work on classification and description of psychiatric disorders, Kraepelin distinguished between dementia praecox and depressions primarily on the basis of outcome.[4] He further divided depressions into two main groups—involutional melancholic and manic-depressive illness—and, in doing so, instituted the view that depressions could be classified.

He distinguished between these two major groups on the basis of limited symptom criteria, age of onset, and family history. Involutional melancholia was characterized by agitation, delusions of guilt, and onset in middle age. Manic-depressive illness included a classic type as well as several heterogeneous and rather dissimilar disorders—all of which were often difficult to reconcile. The classic prototype was characterized by periodicity, weight loss, psychomotor retardation, positive family history for the disorder, and the absence of external precipitants (i.e., it was endogenous). The issue of precipitants, however, became a confusing one in Kraepelin's system since he noted that some manic-depressive states might indeed be precipitated. Further, under the heading of manic-depressive illness, he subsumed psychogenic depressions which represented reactions to environmental stress. At first, these were viewed as having similar symptoms to the classic state; however, Kraepelin noted later that symptoms in these states were reactive (i.e., varied with environmental input) in contrast to more stable symptoms in the classic state.[5] Thus, Kraepelin created an endogenous/exogenous dichotomy which, although given great diagnostic significance, was not hard and fast and later became a source of confusion.

Other areas of confusion which emerged from Kraepelin were the relationships between neuroses, psychoses, and affective disorders. Kraepelin used the term *psychotic* to describe manic-depressive illness, noting that even if delusions were absent the term nevertheless reflected potential for suicide. Thus began multiple defining of *psychotic* in regard to affective disorders, whereas *psychotic* has now come to signify a disorder of severe proportions as well as a thought disorder or break with reality. Kraepelin also implied a linkage between endogenous and psychotic, setting forth a European tradition to use the terms synonymously. Further confusion also resulted from Kraepelin's subsuming neurotic and neurasthenic states under manic-depressive illness, implying the former were variants of the latter.

In summary, Kraepelin's pioneer work in the differentiation and classification of psychiatric disorders separated manic-depressive from involutional melancholia, providing definite but limited criteria for both. However, he generated some controversy regarding the inclusion of most depressions under manic-depressive illness, the significance of precipitants (endogenous vs. exogenous), and the use of the terms *neurotic* and *psychotic* and their relationship.

Shortly thereafter, Lange attempted to clarify and to elaborate Kraepelin's work and divided the continuum of manic-depressive illness into three major groups: classic nonprecipitated disorder (endogenous), "psychogenic melancholia" (exogenous), and an intermediary (mixed) group.[18] He elaborated further on criteria for diagnosis and differentiated between the endogenous and exogenous poles on several counts: "reactivity," symptoms, and family history. The endogenous type was nonprecipitated and its symptoms were not influenced by the environment. Primary symptoms included psychomotor retardation, self-reproach, weight loss, dryness of mouth, and constipation. Family history was positive for manic-depressive illness. Exogenous depressions, however, were characterized by reactivity of symptoms, relative absence of vegetative signs, a tendency to blame the environment, and a family history for schizophrenia, epilepsy, or constitutional psychopathy. Although Lange proposed differences in symptoms, he noted that they were often quite subtle and perhaps failed to discriminate between types of disorders. This may in part have reflected the relative inadequacy of statistical tools at that time which limited one's ability to demonstrate significant differences. In addition, Lange elaborated on the reactivity dimension as having particular diagnostic significance. In Lange's work, reactivity begins to become firmly linked with precipitation (i.e., reactivity of symptoms becomes linked with the existence of precipitating causes), and, as I will attempt to show in this chapter, later works often confused these rather separate dimensions.

Further, one must note that Lange's work defines exogenous symptoms primarily as the absence of endogenous ones. This lack of positive symptom criteria for exogenous states becomes an important area of debate since one was easily led to argue that exogenous states could not be clearly defined by themselves.

Across the channel, the debate was considerably more heated as some workers emphasized an endogenous/exogenous dichotomy while others favored a unitary theory. As noted previously, Mapother believed that depression was a unitary disorder and argued against subclassification.[1] He also reaffirmed Kraepelin's inclusion of neurotic states under affective illness.

Sir Aubrey Lewis, in 1934, in a work which has become a classic, also argued that depressive disorders represented variations of a unitary (rather than binary) disorder.[6] Studying in detail some sixty cases, he found that precipitants and other characteristics did not distinguish between disorders and proposed that all depressive disorders were a variation of a single illness. He did not deny that subtypes existed but emphasized a then-current inability to demonstrate clearly clinical differences. Differences were felt primarily to represent variations in degree rather than in type of illness.

Gillespie (1929),[11] avoiding the use of manic-depressive illness as a major heading, proposed a triadic classification for depression: reactive, autonomous, and involutional. The description of involutional melancholia was similar to Kraepelin's and the remainder of this system bore great similarity to Lange's with *reactive* and *autonomous* corresponding to *exogenous* and *endogenous*. In Gillespie's system, these groups were differentiated on the basis of reactivity, premorbid personality, symptoms, and family history. Gillespie agreed with Lange on the significance of reactivity of symptoms, blame of environment, and retardation as differentiating criteria but disagreed on the role of precipitants and on the significance of other symptoms.

Premorbid personalities of reactive depressives were quiet and shy. When depressed, these patients were often anxious and some appeared more neurotic than depressed. Gillespie, however, emphasized the primacy of their affective illness. It must be noted that the diagnosis of reactive depression and its relationship to characterologic and neurotic disorders has been an area of continuous debate since Gillespie's time.

Autonomous depressions did not vary with environmental stimuli and were characterized by self-accusation, positive family history, and vigorous/ambitious premorbid personalities. Subsumed under this group were: schizophrenia depressions, manic-depressive illness, depressions which were a "further development of a personality," and others not further classified.

Much of Gillespie's work has become an integral part of later systems. Of particular significance were the demarcation of symptom criteria especially in regard to endogenous types, the position that precipitating factors were nondiscriminating, the use of the term *autonomous,* and the inclusion of schizophrenia-related depressions.

Buzzard[19] used the terms *neurotic* and *psychotic* to depict the two major poles of depression which Lange had termed *exogenous* and *endogenous* and Gillespie *reactive* and *autonomous*. Buzzard supported some of their positions but refuted others. He differentiated the two groups by reactivity of symptoms (present in neurotic patients and absent in psychotic ones); presence of vegetative signs and symptoms in psychotic patients but their absence in neurotic ones; self-blame in psychotic depressions and blame of others in neurotic states; and positive family history of suicide and alcoholism in patients with psychotic disorders. Buzzard, however, de-emphasized sleep disturbance in psychotic disorders. Also, precipitants were not proposed as differentiating criteria. Overall, Buzzard linked neurotic depressions, reactivity, and the absence of vegetative signs on the one hand and, on the other, psychotic depression, autonomous states, and the presence of vegetative signs. Again, symptoms of neurotic depressions primarily were defined negatively, i.e., as the absence of those found in psychotic counterparts.

In Europe, early writings reflected pioneer efforts in understanding and classifying the morass of psychiatric disorders. With increased study and demarcation came considerable debate, first revolving primarily around the unitary and binary approaches. Within the binary approach, controversy emerged as to grouping of criteria and definition of terms. For example, Gillespie and Buzzard agreed on reactivity, retardation, and direction of blame as differentiating criteria but differed on the significance of precipitants, various vegetative symptoms, and labels for syndromes. In general, positive symptom criteria for the nonendogenous states were not defined. The varying findings, emphases, and uses of terms presented some confusion to later workers, particularly in regard to the varying linkage of discrete dimensions—symptoms, reactivity, precipitants, and psychosis—to denote either severity or a break with reality.

Later Writings

By the 1950s, psychiatric research had become influenced greatly by technological advances, particularly the computer analysis of data. Investigators began to apply the computer to study groups of depressed patients. Their goal was to establish classification by showing significant differences between subgroups in the distribution of a host of symptoms and characteristics. The debate thus took on a new appearance, although it continued to revolve around many of the same issues. Further, the development of effective treatments—antidepressants and electroconvulsive treatment (ECT)—provided a new incentive to refine classifications further.

Hamilton and White subdivided a number of depressed patients, on the basis of presence or absence of precipitants, into four groups: two distinct poles—endogenous and reactive—and two intermediary groups—doubtful endogenous and doubtful reactive.[7] Thereafter, an inventory of symptoms (Hamilton Scale)[20] was applied to the patients and statistically significant differences were demonstrated between the endogenous and reactive groups on four items in addition to precipitation, which was shown to be a discriminating variable. More specifically, endogenous depressions were marked by more frequent presence of depressed mood, loss of insight, psychomotor retardation, guilt, early-morning awakening, and suicidal ideation. In contrast, the authors were not able to demonstrate any positive characteristics, other than precipitants, which were more frequently present in the reactive group. Several explanations can be proposed for this phenomenon: the limited number of characteristics studied; the study chiefly of characteristics commonly associated with the endogenous state; the possible absence of unique criteria; and the heterogeneity of reactive states, which may include neurotic and other disorders. At any rate, this study began to suggest statistically the possibility that endogenous states had rather definite symptoms and were more homogeneous than their reactive counterparts. Further, distribution of scores suggested a bimodal, dichotomous distribution which others have felt would have been clearer had the sample been larger.

Kiloh and Garside employed factor analysis to study a large sample of depressed patients whom they categorized into endogenous or neurotic types whenever possible.[2] They substituted the term *neurotic* for *reactive*, noting the term *reactive* was confusing since it described two separate characteristics: precipitants and variation with environmental stimuli. Using an inventory, which was more comprehensive than the Hamilton Scale and which included symptoms as well as other critieria, they were able to demonstrate a bipolar factor of characteristics which corresponded to an endogenous/neurotic dichotomy. They were able to define positive criteria for both endogenous and neurotic depressions. Endogenous depressions were characterized by, among others, early-morning awakening, depression being worse in morning, retardation, duration of present illness of one year or less, failure of concentration, weight loss, and history of previous attacks. Neurotic depressions, on the other hand, were noted by their reactivity of symptoms, precipitation, self-pity, variability of illness, hysterical features, initial insomnia, depression being worse in evening, hypochondriasis, and obsessionality.

The authors proposed applications for their classification since they believed in the importance of proper diagnosis and classification to determine appropriate treatment. This study was an extension of earlier work in which response to imipramine correlated positively with endogenous symptoms and negatively with neurotic ones.[21] Subsequently, this group was also able to demonstrate similar findings for ECT response.[22] Thus, classification had begun to take on a significance which had not been possible at the time of Mapother and others.

Although the work of Kiloh and Garside supported a clear endogenous/neurotic dichotomy, it did not avoid later controversy and continued some previous confusion. The work confirmed an association between precipitation and reactivity, an issue which has remained in some debate. An additional murky area in this work is the use of the term *neurotic.* Although their neurotic depressive patients did show more in the way of obsessionality and hysteria, the term *neurotic* is not really defined. It implies a relationship between a type of depression and the neuroses again leading to a confusion of terms. Kendell[8] has noted that many European investigators have used *neurotic* synonymously with *reactive* to indicate a less severe disorder, often characterized by anxiety, self-pity, and histrionics, while North Americans have defined *neurotic* more narrowly to indicate primarily the absence of a break with reality, distinguishing it from both psychotic and reactive states. Ascher, in this country, has criticized the use of neurotic to indicate merely a mild disorder.[23]

In the United States, several workers have proposed that endogenous depressions represent only one of several possible subtypes of depressive disorders. Thus, the endogenous reactive dichotomy came to be viewed as but one aspect of a larger classification system. This was consistent with the work of some American and European workers who have emphasized a pluralistic classification of depressive disease, perhaps most graphic in DSMII of the American Psychiatric Association.

Employing factor analysis of data collected on a sample of depressed patients, Rosenthal (working with both Klerman and Gudeman) has demonstrated the existence of endogenous and nonendogenous factors. Rosenthal and Klerman[17] proposed a triad of characteristics for endogenous depressions: (1) particular pattern of manifest symptoms (similar to those noted in other studies); (2) well-adjusted, nonneurotic premorbid personality; (3) less frequent precipitants and nonreactive symptoms. Rosenthal and Gudeman,[24] in a later study, confirmed these findings noting, however, that premorbid obsessional traits were not uncommon in endogenously depressed patients. They proposed the term *autonomous* be substituted for *endogenous* since symptoms of the endogenous pattern are not reactive to environmental stimuli, and endogenous states may often be precipitated, albeit less frequently. This de-emphasis of precipitants has achieved increasing popularity since precipitants are often difficult to define and life stresses can precede depressions of the endogenous type. The importance of these works rests with the proposal that the endogenous pattern was but one subtype of depression and could be defined on the basis of symptoms, autonomy, and well-adjusted premorbid personality rather than on the lack of precipitants. However, the notion that endogenous states occurred only in patients with relatively healthy premorbid personalities has become a source of later debate.

In a subsequent paper, Rosenthal and Gudeman[25] presented data supporting the existence of a second factor—corresponding to a nonendogenous syndrome termed the *self-pitying constellation*. The five symptoms which loaded positively for it (i.e., were often present) included:

hypochrondriasis, psychic anxiety, demanding and complaining behavior, self-pity, and somatic anxiety. Less frequently present were hostility, fatigue, weight loss, and early evening insomnia. This factor was noted by negative loading (frequent absence) of retardation, guilt, suicidal symptoms, worthlessness, and paranoid ideation. The authors drew parrallels between their findings and those particularly of Kiloh and Garside.[2] However, Kendell subsequently noted that, taken as a whole, writings on endogenous states appear to describe many different subtypes.[8]

Of particular importance were the authors' findings that some items loaded positively for one group or the other, some loaded positively for both, and others negatively for both. Further, some patients demonstrated combinations of both factors, such that two were not mutually exclusive groups into which all depressed patients could be divided. This then argued against the view that all depressions could be divided clearly into an endogenous or a nonendogenous group.

A source of confusion which begins to emerge from the work of Rosenthal et al. is an emphasis on a well-adjusted predisposition for diagnosing endogenous depressions. This may have great implication for the practitioner. Overemphasis on a healthy predisposition may lead to underdiagnosing endogenous depressions and overdiagnosing neurotic ones, particularly if the subject has a history of neurotic symptoms. This could then lead to practitioners' finding a more homogeneous endogenous group and a larger, heterogeneous neurotic group. In addition, rigid and varying criteria for the neurotic depressions might lead to a small number of such patients and a query as to their existence. Further, a well-adjusted predisposition may be misleading since such patients may mask psychological conflicts which can be quite limiting although clinically undiagnosable. (See Chapter 9 by Isenberg and Schatzberg.) The end result would be an erroneous, dichotomous classification since patients may have premorbid (possibly neurotic) conflicts and still develop endogenous depressions.

Kendell has noted that, although most later workers have demonstrated a core set of symptoms which corresponded to an endogenous syndrome, some have failed to replicate a clear boundary line between endogenous and nonendogenous depressions.[13,15] Rather, these workers have proposed a dimensional approach based on an endogenous–neurotic continuum. Part of the difficulty in replicating a dichotomy has been felt to be methodological, and the reader is referred elsewhere for a discussion of some of the issues.[8,26] Of note, however, is that Eysenck[26] has maintained that workers have often confused two separate issues in classification (unitary vs. binary and categorical vs. dimensional) and this confusion has limited some workers' ability to demonstrate a dichotomy. Eysenck argued further that factor-analytic study of symptoms has resulted in clear dichotomies but that two separate dimensions were needed to describe patients. Thus, he favored a binary, dimensional approach and proposed that two orthogonal dimensions—neuroticism and psychoticism—be applied to each subject.

In spite of Eysenck's work, the endogenous/nonendogenous debate has continued. Part of the confusion has stemmed from an inability to define a homogeneous nonendogenous state. Although there is evidence for a group of disorders which differs from the endogenous type in the absence of vegetative signs, in reactivity of symptoms, in possible precipitants, and in the presence of neurotic and characterologic traits, this second group appears to be more diffuse, to have been variously defined, and to include possibly a host of depressive, neurotic, or personality disorders. Some workers have gone so far as to argue that the second group may not reflect a depressive disorder and thus cannot be separated clearly from endogenous states under one umbrella of depression (i.e., an argument against a clear endogenous/reactive dichotomy). More specifically, Mendels and others[12,27] have postulated that endogenous depressions represent the classic depressive syndrome while reactive states are mixed disorders in which depression is but one factor, and McConaghy et al.[16] claimed that neurotic depressions reflected nonspecific reactions in patients with premorbid personality disorders. The issue today is still moot and, as we will show, recent workers (e.g., Klein and Schildkraut) have again proposed symptoms and other criteria for the nonendogenous syndromes. In summary, the literature supports an endogenous type of depressive disorder but the description and classification of nonendogenous counterparts is open to some debate as is their relationship to an endogenous syndrome.

OTHER FACTOR-ANALYTIC STUDIES

Several workers who employed factor analysis to study depressed patients proposed alternate systems which did not include a clear endogenous/nonendogenous dichotomy. A major example of such an approach is the extensive study by Grinker et al.[28] They were able to cluster certain symptoms and behaviors in a group of depressed patients and to identify four pure subgroups into which some 40% of their patients could be clearly divided. Two sets of distinct criteria—feelings and behavior—were proposed for each group. In addition, they postulated constellations of dynamics, ego defenses, and treatment responses which might correspond to the groups.

Pattern A was felt "close to the common stereotype of depression" and was characterized by feelings of hopelessness, loss of self-esteem, and some guilt. Behavior was characterized by withdrawal, isolation, apathy, slowing of speech and thinking, and cognitive disturbance. These patients were also characterized by the absence of hypochondriasis, anxiety, clinging and love-seeking behavior, and many somatic symptoms.

Pattern B patients were characterized by feelings of dismal hopelessness, low self-esteem, considerable guilt, and great anxiety. Behavior was characterized by agitation and clinging demands for attention. There was a relative absence of slowed speech, impaired thinking, hypochondriasis, and psychosomatic symptoms.

Pattern C was characterized by a feeling of not being loved but by less-than-average depressed affect, guilt, and anxiety. Behavior was primarily agitated, demanding, and hypochondriacal, and there were also psychosomatic symptoms. Although they complained irrationally, these patients showed relatively little dismal and hopeless affect. The investigators felt the picture suggested that of the hypochondriac who may have a history of schizoid or borderline traits.

Pattern D was characterized by feelings of gloom, hopelessness, anxiety, and some guilt. However, they did not cling or demand attention. Behavior was characterized by demanding, provocative acts. These people were not withdrawn, not continually seeking attention, nor were they hypochondriacal. Patients in this group were termed *angry depressives*. Premorbidly, they had been narcissistic and highly aggressive and their illness often resulted from their becoming unable to dominate their environment.

Overall et al. applied the Brief Psychiatric Rating Scale (BPRS) to a group of depressed patients.[29] Employing factor analysis of results of this scale, they were able to identify three groups: anxious–tense depression, hostile depression, and retarded depression. The anxious–tense group was the largest and was characterized by anxiety and depression; patients in this group were often diagnosed as neurotic or reactive depressions. The hostile depression group was characterized by great irritability—often in conjunction with some agitation. The last group, retarded depression, appeared to correspond to a clear, endogenous type. This system was felt to have clinical significance since, in this study, anxiously depressed patients tended to respond to thioridazine while their retarded, depressed counterparts tended to respond to imipramine.

PLURALISTIC SYSTEMS AND DSMI AND II

Early pluralistic systems are perhaps most clearly associated with the work of Adolph Meyer, who proposed that psychiatric disorders represented individualistic reactions to internal or external stresses. The work of Meyer undoubtedly supported the notion that some depressions are precipitated. Muncie's[30] 1939 textbook, based greatly on Meyerian principles, subdivides depressive reactions (thymergasia) into several subtypes, all of which were subsumed under holergasias or major psychotic reactions. A primary criterion for the major reactions was the patient's committability, which by the author's own admission was difficult to determine. This work is not devoid of many of the confusions noted previously—more specifically, the significance of environmental precipitants and the multiple uses of the term *psychotic*. Some of these confusions have been carried over into both DSMs of the APA. DSMI, published in 1952,[31] clearly demonstrated Meyer's influence since most disorders were termed *reactive* (i.e., *precipitated*) and most depressions were subsumed under psychosis. At that time, little was known about somatic therapies for particular types of depression (let alone biology, genetics, and outcome) and there was a greater emphasis on psychotherapy as a primary treatment modality in depression and other disorders.

DSMII[32] was developed at a time when more was becoming known about the treatment of depression; however, knowledge of genetics, family history, and biology was still limited. DSMII is outlined in Table I.

In this classification, differentiation is often based on severity and precipitants rather than symptoms. Major affective disorders are subsumed under psychoses as are the schizophrenias. Looking more closely, one notes again that psychosis has various meanings. For

TABLE I. DSMII CLASSIFICATION OF DEPRESSIVE DISORDERS

- I. Psychoses not attributed to physical conditions
  - A. Schizophrenia
    - 1. Schizoaffective type
  - B. Major affective disorders
    - 1. Involutional melancholia
    - 2. Manic-depressive illness
      - (a) manic type
      - (b) depressed type
      - (c) circular type
  - C. Other psychoses
    - 1. Psychotic depressive reaction
- II. Neuroses
  - A. Depressive neurosis

schizophrenia, it is used primarily to designate a thought disorder or distortion in reality testing, the more traditional meaning. For affective disorders, psychosis also denotes an inability to function in one's environment, implying a more severe illness in contrast to a mild or neurotic disorder. Since the DSMII provides rather limited symptom criteria for psychotic depressive reaction and neurotic depression, differentiation between the two at times becomes based on severity (rather than impairment of reality testing)—a state of affairs suggested by Lewis some 40 years ago. The system also dictates that manic depressions are psychotic either because they are severe in intensity or accompanied by delusions or hallucinations. Clearly, this is a misleading dictum.

Confusion also stems from the reliance on precipitating events as criteria for classification. The DSMII distinguishes between psychotic-depressive reaction and depressive neurosis, on the one hand, and manic-depressive illness on the other. The former are precipitated by events; the latter is not. Symptoms of psychotic-depressive reaction and manic-depressive illness, depressed state, may be similar and include primarily severely depressed mood and psychomotor retardation. Other symptoms may include apprehension, perplexity, and anxiety. Thus, two patients with similar symptoms of severe retardation would be diagnosed differently (i.e., manic-depressive, depressed-state, or psychotic-depressive reaction) solely because of precipitating events. This is a problem since manic-depressive states may be preceded by an important event and thus patients would be misdiagnosed.

Further, manic-depressive illness in this system appears to include a possible heterogeneous group of disorders as it subsumes nonprecipitated, severe depressions with no history of previous manic attacks. It is indeed probable—as will be cited later—that the occurrence of mania may be a significant differentiating criterion and that patients who demonstrate retarded depressions, without a positive history of mania, may not be manic-depressive.

Last, DSMII lists involutional melancholia separately from manic-depressive illness, although it notes that it may actually be a subtype. Kendell has noted that several workers in recent years have indicated that involutional melancholia may be a variation of unipolar depression which can occur at other ages in addition to the "classic" age of onset.[8,33]

To summarize, DSMII defines and subdivides depressive states in a rather limited way. Several separate dimensions appear to be confused, and there is a trend toward some unnecessary rigidity in criteria for classification (e.g., nonprecipitation of manic-depressive states). The result is a classification that is confusing and at times difficult to apply. For example, difficulty arises when one attempts to apply it to diagnose a manic-depressive patient (with a history of mania) who appears mildly depressed and retarded but remains in contact with reality. Many would call him manic-depressive, but in DSMII this would mean a nonfunctional, psychotic state without precipitants. However, the patient is not psychotic, he can work, and his illness has been precipitated by an external event. Depressive neurosis does not appear to be a suitable category, particularly in view of the previous history. It is important to note that DSMII is in the process of revision and many of these issues are being discussed with an eye toward revamping the system in an attempt to make it more applicable. (See Addendum, p. 37.)

NEWER RESEARCH SYSTEMS

In the 1960s and 1970s, researchers working in various areas of affective disease began to use data on age of onset, course, treatment response, genetics, and biology to improve upon the classification of depressive disorders. As early as 1959, Leonhard[34] proposed that manic-depressive illness be divided into two groups; bipolar (alternating mania and depression) and unipolar (recurrence in one state without the other). A few years later, this dichotomy proved to be valid as differences were demonstrated between the two groups in age of onset, length and frequency of episodes, and family history.[35] Kendell has noted that today this differentiation is generally agreed upon. However, since depressive symptoms may be identical in both groups, the diagnosis in an initial episode is difficult. Some patients who are initially diagnosed as unipolar may eventually become hypomanic, necessitating a change in diagnosis to bipolar. Our group has been working on methods to differentiate between unipolar and bipolar depressives on the basis of catecholamine excretion in the urine. (See Chapter 3 by Schildkraut et al.) The differentiation between unipolar and bipolar disorders is extremely important clinically since lithium carbonate may prove to be more effective than tricyclics as prophylaxis in the bipolar disorders.[36] (See Chapter 8 by Cole.)

St. Louis System

In an attempt to provide ways of including family history and outcome data, the St. Louis group has developed a classification system for psychiatric disorders which is based fundamentally on symptoms and history.[37–39] The overall system is intended to provide research criteria for diagnosis and study of psychiatric disorders and is based on a study of a group of mixed psychiatric patients. Included is a limited classification of affective disorders which provides criteria for the diagnosis of depressions and mania. The St. Louis group proposed five criteria for classification of diseases: clinical description, laboratory studies, exclusion of other syndromes, family studies, and follow-up.[39]

In their system, schizophrenia and primary affective disease are mutually exclusive—i.e., a patient can be diagnosed either but not both. The system divides depressive disorders into two major groups: primary and secondary.[38,39] Unlike many others, this group has sought to distinguish depressive mood from a depressive episode, primarily on the basis of specific symptoms. An episode lasts at least one month and is defined as a depressive mood in conjunction with at least five of the following somatic or vegetative signs: poor appetite, sleep difficulty, loss of energy, agitation or retardation, guilt, decreased ability to think, suicidal ideation, and decreased interest in activities.[39] An important feature is the proposal that diagnosis be based on the presence of a minimal core of symptoms extracted from a larger group. This implies a variability of the disorder and militates against too rigid a classification.

The St. Louis system distinguishes between primary and secondary depressions on the basis of history and outcome. Primary depressions are depressive episodes occurring in patients with no previous psychiatric history other than that of affective disorders. Secondary depressions are episodes occurring in patients with a definite preexisting psychiatric illness, including among others: "organic brain syndromes," anxiety, neurosis, antisocial personality, and homosexuality. Also, patients with depressions occurring in the context of a severe physical illness are considered "secondary." However, in this approach, many possible secondary depressive patients did not fulfill the necessary criteria for other personality-type disorders and were placed in an undiagnosed group. This may reflect diagnostic criteria which are too stringent for these disorders.[38] Finally, the investigators noted that this system had not further subdivided the depressive disorders into categories.[39]

Winokur

Winokur, who worked with the St. Louis group, elaborated on their system[40] and proposed a system which was based in large part on family or genetic studies and which further subdivided depressive disorders. The system is outlined in Table II. As in the St. Louis system, all groups in Winokur's system required lowered mood along with a cluster of possible vegetative signs. Autonomy was not included as a criterion.

Grief reaction was proposed as a model for reactive states since such patients demonstrate vegetative symptoms and improve over a 6- to 10-week period. The primary and secondary depressions were similar to the St. Louis definition and criteria for mania are also provided. Depressed patients with a family history of mania are listed under manic-depressive. Two groups were elucidated for unipolar depressions—primarily on the basis of differences in family history. Pure depressive disease was more common in men and was associated with a family history of affective disease in first-degree relatives. Depression spectrum disease was most common in women with a high incidence of depression, alcoholism, and sociopathy in first-degree relatives.

TABLE II. WINOKUR CLASSIFICATION OF DEPRESSIVE DISORDERS

I. Grief state—model for reactive depression
II. Secondary depression
III. Primary affective disorder
  A. Manic-depressive
    1. Clinical picture of mania and depression
    2. Clinical picture of depression only but family history of mania
  B. Depressive disease (unipolar)
    1. Pure
    2. Spectrum disorder

The Winokur system poses several problems. First, as in the St. Louis system, it defines uniformly all depressions primarily in terms of somatic symptoms, without regard to autonomy, and does not attempt to distinguish between endogenous and nonendogenous types. Instead, it implies that nonendogenous depressions are either not primarily depressed, reflect extensions of other disorders, or do not exist. Thus it does not allow for patients who were described by such previous workers as Rosenthal and Gudeman[25] or Kiloh and Garside.[2] Second, by introducing the issue of precipitants and reactive depressions (i.e., grief reaction) without regard to symptom differences, it again raises the question as to the significance of events in the etiology of depressive episodes and their relationship to symptom variations. It must be noted that Winokur is tentative in introducing grief as a model for reactive states, and indeed further study is necessary to define both its symptoms and its relationship to other types of depressions. As I will discuss later Klein and Schildkraut propose rather different symptom criteria for such reactions. Further, the dichotomy between primary and secondary affective disease is open to question, requires further study, and may not be justified. For example, while manic-depressive patients often show no previous history of psychiatric illness, the occurrence of other diseases—particularly alcoholism—is not without possibility.[41] However, in both Winokur's and the St. Louis system, such rather classic, bipolar patients would be diagnosed as having a secondary affective disorder. Last, the classification of depressed patients with a family history of mania as manic-depressive requires further study and validation.

Klein

Klein has recently proposed a system that includes an endogenous–nonendogenous dichotomy and provides criteria for both groups.[42] Klein's system is based on clinical experience with depressed patients, particularly their response to tricyclics. The system provides a proposed method for predicting which patients will respond to the tricyclic, imipramine, and thus has relevance to clinical management. Depressive disorders are divided into three major groups: endogenomorphic, acute dysphoria (reactive), and chronic overreactive dysphoria (neurotic). Endogenomorphic depression is precipitated in less than half the cases and is characterized primarily by an inhibition in ability to experience pleasure. Other symptoms include many of those proposed by others for endogenous depressions and those proposed by the St. Louis group for both their groups. As in Winokur's system, Klein's endogenomorphic group can further be divided into unipolar and bipolar types according to history. Regarding treatment, Klein has postulated that tricyclics work primarily on central pleasure centers: thus, the group is highly responsive to tricyclics and resistant to placebo.

On the other hand, the capacity for experiencing pleasure generally remains intact in both nonendogenomorphic groups, which Klein notes may ultimately prove to be subdivisions of one continuous group. Klein's chronic overreactive dysphoria is precipitated in half the cases and is characterized by anger and demoralization. The disorder represents a "chronic overreaction to disappointment," and Klein uses the term *neurotic* as a qualifying adjective. These patients do poorly on placebo or tricyclics. Acute (reactive) dysphoria represents a reaction to an overwhelming stress in a patient with a previously normal history. Symptoms include feelings of incompetency and dependency. This group shows good response to both placebo and tricyclics. It must be noted that Klein's system provides for sequential expression of symptoms and crossover, such that various admixtures of symptoms are possible. Finally, this system will require further study to validate and support both the basic suppositions and criteria for diagnosis. One issue which may require further elaboration is how differential response of some endogenous-type depressive disorders to amitriptyline rather than to imipramine fits into the system. This differential response correlates with catecholamine excretion and may have implications for classification of depressive disorders as is discussed in the next section.

Schildkraut System

Schildkraut has proposed a comprehensive system which includes among others schizophrenia-related and nonendogenous depressions.[41,43] The system has been developed in conjunction with research on catecholamine execretion patterns as a basis for predicting response to specific tricyclics and for classifying depressive disorders. (See Chapter 3 by Schildkraut et al.) Criteria for diagnosis in this system are based primarily on core systems and overall history. Since the factor-analytic study of symptoms has not been completed, the system at present represents only an applicable research strategy. Depressions are divided into three major groups and then are further subdivided. One area of possible confusion is the provision of criteria for a general syndrome in addition to the specific subtypes. A lack of precipitants is not needed for making the diagnosis of an endogenous state. Most of the depressive subtypes in the system are felt to be endogenous in nature except for chronic characterologic and nonspecific reactions. However, the exact relationship between syndrome diagnosis and clinical subtypes is not entirely clear, particularly since *endogenous* is used in two ways: a general syndrome description and a clinical subtype of unipolar depression. Last, *psychotic* is used only as an adjective to describe a break with reality.

The system, which is outlined in Table III, may be viewed as a decision tree with diagnosis obtained by one's going down the table. One strength of this system rests with its comprehensive classification of schizophrenia-related depressions. Although some 50 years ago Gillespie[11] noted that schizophrenic depressions were a subgroup of "auton-

Table III. Schildkraut Classification of Depressive Disorders

I. Schizophrenia-related depressions
   A. Schizoid-related
   B. Schizophreniform
   C. True or process schizophrenia
II. Bipolar manic-depressive depressions
III. Unipolar depressions
   A. Endogenous
   B. Agitated involutional
   C. Chronic characterologic
   D. Nonspecific syndromes–situational, other

omous" disorders, many subsequent systems have not included or divided them. In fact, some have made a clear distinction between schizophrenia and primary affective disorders. Here, schizophrenia-related depressions are divided into three groups. The first category is "schizoid-related"—a depressive episode occurring in a schizoid disorder. The latter is defined as a history of chronic asocial, bizarre, or eccentric behavior of several years' duration in the absence of a history of psychotic episodes. Schizophreniform depressions are depressions in patients with a history of affect-non-consonant psychotic episodes (including micropsychoses) in the absence of a history of schizoid behavior. True or process schizophrenia is characterized by a thought disorder (represented by signs other than a disturbance in rate of thought and speech), affect-non-consonant delusions or hallucinations, and a history of chronic asocial behavior.

The diagnosis of manic-depressive (bipolar) states requires a positive history of hypomania or mania. In a manner similar to that of the St. Louis and Winokur systems, hypomania is characterized by the presence of several of the following symptoms: pressure of speech, flight of ideas, increased sense of vitality, euphoria, grandiosity, irritability, acceleration, intrusiveness, increased spending of money, and decreased need for sleep. Mania is defined as hypomania in combination with unresponsiveness to verbal command or destructiveness.

Unipolar depressions occur in those depressed patients who do not have histories of schizophrenia-related or bipolar disorders. They may then be further divided into one of four groups, of which endogenous and chronic characterologic (nonendogenous) syndromes represent the two major ones. At the core of this system is the observation that patients rarely demonstrate both syndromes simultaneously. Differentiation between groups is based primarily on fulfilling minimum core symptoms, which differ for the two major groups. Overall history, though important, is secondary. As in the St. Louis system, requiring a minimum rather than an absolute set of symptoms militates against too rigid a classification and allows for variation. Endogenous depressions are characterized by adequate premorbid functioning and autonomous symptoms, including psychic retardation, loss of energy, decreased initiative, anhedonia, and diurnal variation (depression worse in morning). These symptoms are similar to those presented in other systems. Precipitants may or may not be present in these states. Secondary symptoms which are commonly but not necessarily present include sadness, sleep disturbance, anorexia, feelings of hopelessness and helplessness, decreased self-esteem, guilt and remorse, demoralization, and suicidal ruminations. These symptoms may be present in chronic characterologic depressives as well and thus do not represent primary distinguishing factors.

Involutional melancholia is characterized by those symptoms seen in endogenous states; however, agitation (pacing and other behaviors) and delusions of a paranoid, guilty, or bodily nature may also be prominent. While most patients are middle-aged, the syndrome may occur in younger age groups. Although this group is listed separately, Schildkraut has also suggested that it may reflect an endogenous subtype. These observations are in line with the works of others who have felt it was a unipolar variant.[8,33,44] In addition, as illustrated previously, recent classifications (such as the St. Louis, Winokur, and Klein) have not included it as a separate entity. The issue, however, is by no means settled and further work will be required to resolve it.

Distinguishing signs and symptoms of the chronic characterologic syndrome include unhappiness, tearfulness or tendency to weep, dissatisfaction, histrionic and dramatic behavior, clinging dependency, responsivity of symptoms to environmental stimuli, pessimism, anger/irritability, anxiety, and preoccupation with illness. These patients often (but not necessarily) have lifelong difficulties in dealing with interpersonal relationships and "minor stress may precipitate symptomatology."

They may demonstrate manipulative and suicidal behavior, secondary gain, and the misuse of alcohol and other drugs. Overall, the group probably contains may heterogeneous syndromes. Some might argue that they represent personality rather than affective disorders; however, such patients demonstrate significantly lowered mood and sadness. In this system, use of the term *chronic characterologic* is misleading since patients may not have characterologic problems nor are their illnesses necessarily chronic.

Situational depressive syndromes represent a reaction to an overpowering stress such as a loss of a close relative. Primary symptoms include tearfulness, brooding, preoccupation with precipitating factor, anxiety, anorexia, and sleep disturbance. The state is reactive to environmental stimuli, so that during these episodes the patient may still experience some pleasure. Symptoms in this disorder may evolve into those seen in an autonomous or endogenous disorder, and in that case the diagnosis would be changed. This group differs from Winokur's grief reaction in that symptoms provided are not those of a more typical endogenous state.

A significant aspect of this research revolves around the potential use of biological measures (e.g., urinary excretion of catecholamine metabolites and platelet monoamine oxidase activity) and response to tricyclics to classify patients. As illustrated in the chapter by Schildkraut et al., patients with manic-depressive depressions may be separated from chronic characterologic depressions on the basis of a profile of urinary catecholamine metabolites including MHPG (3-methoxy-4-hydroxyphenylglycol), which is relatively low in bipolar depressions and high in chronic characterologic ones. By extension, the diagnosis of potentially manic patients via urine excretion study would provide a way for defining a population at risk and for instituting early preventive treatment. Further, several workers have shown that high MHPG execretion correlates with amitriptyline response,[45,46] while low MHPG execretion correlates with imipramine response.[46,47] Maas[48] has postulated two types of depressive illness. One is characterized by low MHPG execretion, a disorder in norepinephrine metabolism, normal serotonin "activity," and response to imipramine. The other is characterized by high MHPG excretion, "normal" norepinephrine activity, disorder in serotonin metabolism, and response to amitriptyline. (See Chapter 2 by Goodwin and Potter.) Thus, this work is hopefully providing methods for ultimately correlating symptoms, history, biology, and treatment of the many depressive disorders.

In summary, Schildkraut's system provides an opportunity to classify in detail many depressive syndromes, including those in schizophrenia-related groups, and, coupled with biochemical study, may prove to be a comprehensive system for classification. Symptom criteria are provided for endogenous and nonendogenous syndromes. Precipitants, however, are not viewed as discriminatory, and *psychotic* is used only to denote a break with reality. Although one may argue that chronic characterologic depressions reflect other types of disorders, their inclusion in a system is useful and probably warranted—if only to support further study. As with some others, this system requires validation and factor analysis of symptom variables.

SUMMARY

Although a great deal of confusion (often semantic) about classification still exists, considerable progress has been made. It appears that the trend is toward a pluralistic, categorical system based fundamentally on symptoms and history. Agreement has emerged on the unipolar/bipolar distinction and the existence of a rather specific endogenous or autonomous state. Also, there is a trend toward viewing involutional depressions as a variant of unipolar illness. The nonendogenous disorders, however, are not agreed upon and may ultimately prove to be truly heterogeneous. Further work is required to sort out this group. One great hope is that advances in research on the genetics, outcome, biochemistry, and treatment response of depressive disorders are beginning to provide important correlates to systems based on symptoms and history. Indeed, some day a universally accepted system may be formulated—one in which patients can be diagnosed as having a specific illness with particular symptoms, specific biological findings, family history, course and outcome, and treatment responsivity. To reach this end, much work will be required, but progress in recent years augurs well for solution of those basic questions which troubled Mapother some 50 years ago.

ADDENDUM—DSMIII

At the time this chapter was originally written, DMSIII was still being developed. However, as this book was being sent to press, DSMIII entered its final stages, and Dr. Robert Spitzer has made available materials for this section. In the new system, all patients will be evaluated along five discrete axes: diagnosis of presenting illness, existing personality characteristics/disorders, contributing physical disorders, level of premorbid functioning, and severity of preceding stressors. By separating various dimensions, this system will enable the practitioner to avoid quagmires previously encountered with DSMII.

In the DSMIII, the affective disorders are distinguished from schizophrenic illnesses and are divided into three major types: episodic, chronic, and atypical. All three are subdivided further into depressive, manic, and bipolar (circular) subtypes. Criteria are provided for what constitutes an episode and include a relatively clear demarcation from adequate premorbid functioning. Coding provides for indicating the total number of episodes. Core operational symptom criteria for episodic subtypes are similar to those proposed in St. Louis', Schildkraut's, and other classifications for hypomanic/manic, endogenous, and primary depressive disorders. Since precipitants are rated along a separate axis and their presence is not a criterion for exclusion from episodic depressive or bipolar disorders, a major stumbling block of DSMII has been overcome. Further, operational criteria are provided for degrees of severity with *psychotic* (indicated only by presence of delusions and hallucinations) implying the greatest severity, a point of possible confusion. Autonomy of syndrome is not a criterion for diagnosis but rather one for moderate severity.

Chronic depressive disorders are by definition not psychotic. Rather, they represent an intermittently occurring depressive disorder lasting hours to days, with intervals of normal mood lasting days to weeks. The syndrome may correspond to a nonendogenous, chronic characterologic, or neurotic depressive disorder. Operational symptom criteria which distinguish it from an episodic disorder include pessimistic attitude, preoccupation with feelings of inadequacy, crying, and brooding about the past. Patients with this disorder commonly may also carry other personality disorder diagnoses. Specific criteria are also provided for the chronic hypomanic and chronic cyclothymic subtypes.

Atypical affective disorders are those which do not meet other criteria. Included in the atypical depressive disorders are chronic-like depressions which are not clearly separable from previous functioning (i.e., not episodic) and have rare symptom-free intervals (i.e., not chronic depressive).

DSMIII also includes two other important depressive disorders: adjustment disorder with depressed mood and schizoaffective disorder, depressed type. Adjustment disorder refers to a depression which does not meet criteria for an episodic depressive disorder and which occurs after major psychosocial stress. Schizoaffective disorders are listed separately from both schizophrenia and affective disorders. Criteria include symptoms for both a depressive episode and a schizophrenic-like syndrome. The latter, however, cannot precede the onset of depression.

Thus, DSMIII, which reflects a major attempt at synthesizing a variety of views, separates dimensions which were previously confused, overcomes many of the stumbling blocks, and provides specific and detailed operational criteria for diagnosis. Possible pitfalls may arise with this system as with others; however, it still promises to be highly usable.

ACKNOWLEDGMENT

This work was supported in part by USPHS Grant No. MH-15413.

REFERENCES

1. Mapother E: Discussion on manic-depressive psychosis. *Br. Med. J. 2*:872–876, 1926.
2. Kiloh LG, Garside RF: The independence of neurotic depression and endogenous depression. *Br. J. Psychiatry 109*:451–463, 1963.
3. Eysenck HJ: Classification and the problems of diagnosis. In: Eysenck HJ (ed) *Handbook of Abnormal Psychology*. London, Pitman, 1960.
4. Kraepelin E: *Lectures on Clinical Psychiatry*. New York, William Wood, 1904.
5. Kraepelin E: *Manic-Depressive Insanity and Paranoia*. Translated by M. Barclay. Edinburgh, E & S Livingstone, 1921.
6. Lewis A: Melancholia: A clinical survey. *J. Ment. Sci. 80*:277–375, 1934.
7. Hamilton M, White JM: Clinical syndromes in depressive states. *J. Ment. Sci. 105*:985–998, 1959.
8. Kendell RE: The classification of depressions: A review of contemporary confusion. *Br. J. Psychiatry 129*:15–28, 1976.
9. Lewis AJ: Melancholia: A historical review. *J. Ment. Sci. 80*:1–42, 1934.
10. Patridge M: Some reflections on the nature of affective disorders arising from the results of prefrontal lobectomy. *J. Ment. Sci. 95*:795–825, 1949.
11. Gillespie RD: The clinical differentiation of types of depression. *Guy's Hosp. Rep. 9*:306–344, 1929.
12. Mendels J, Cochrane C: The nosology of depression: The endogenous reactive concept. *Am. J. Psychiatry 124* (suppl.):1–11, 1968.
13. Kendell RE: *The Classification of Depressive Illnesses*. Maudsley Monograph No. 18. London, Oxford University Press, 1968.
14. Beck AT: *Depression: Causes and Treatment*. Philadelphia, U. of Pennsylvania Press, 1967.
15. Paykel ES, Prusoff B, Klerman GL: The endogenous-neurotic continuum in depression. *J. Psychiat. Res. 8*:73–90, 1971.
16. McConaghy N, Joffe AD, Murphy B: The independence of neurotic and endogenous depression. *Br. J. Psychiatry 113*:479–484, 1964.
17. Rosenthal SH, Klerman GL: Content and consistency in the endogenous depressive pattern. *Br. J. Psychiatry 112*:471–484, 1966.
18. Lange J: Über melancholie. *Z. Neurol. und Psychiat. 101*:293–319, 1926.
19. Buzzard EF: Discussion of the diagnosis and treatment of the milder forms of the manic-depressive psychosis. *Proc. Roy. Soc. Med. 23*:881–883, 1930.
20. Hamilton M: A rating scale for depression. *J. Neurol. Neurosurg. and Psychiatry 23*:56–61, 1960.
21. Kiloh LG, Ball JRB, Garside RF: Prognostic factors in treatment of depressive states with imipramine. *Br. Med. J. 1*:1225–1227, 1962.
22. Carney MWP, Roth M, Garside RF: The diagnosis of depressive syndromes and the prediction of ECT responses. *Br. J. Psychiatry 111*:659–674, 1965.
23. Ascher E: A criticism of the concept of neurotic depression. *Am. J. Psychiatry 108*:901–908, 1952.
24. Rosenthal SH, Gudeman JE: The endogenous depressive pattern. *Arch. Gen. Psychiatry 16*:241–249, 1967.

25. Rosenthal SH, Gudeman JE: The self-pitying constellation in depression. *Br. J. Psychiatry 113:*485–489, 1967.
26. Eysenck HJ: The classification of depressive illness. *Br. J. Psychiatry 117:*241–250, 1970.
27. Mendels J: Depression: The distinction between syndrome and symptom. *Br. J. Psychiatry 114:*1549–1554, 1968.
28. Grinker RR, Miller J, Sabshin M, Nunn R, Nunnally JC: *The Phenomena of Depression.* New York, Paul B. Hueber, 1961.
29. Overall JE, Hollister LE, Johnson M et al. Nosology of depression and differential response to drugs. *JAMA 195:*946–950, 1966.
30. Muncie W: *Psychobiology and Psychiatry.* St. Louis, CV Mosby, 1939.
31. American Psychiatric Association: *Diagnostic and Statistical Manual of Mental Disorders,* ed. I. Washington, DC, 1952.
32. American Psychiatric Association: *Diagnostic and Statistical Manual of Mental Disorders.* ed. II. Washington, DC, 1968.
33. Post F: *The Significance of Affective Symptoms in Old Age.* London, Oxford University Press, 1962.
34. Leonhard K: *Aufteilung der Endogenen Psychosen.* Berlin, Akademie Verlag, 1959.
35. Perris C: A survey of bipolar and unipolar recurrent depressive psychoses. *Acta Psychiat. Scand.* (suppl.):194, 1966.
36. Prien RF, Klett J, Caffey EM: Lithium carbonate and imipramine in prevention of depressive episodes. *Arch. Gen. Psychiatry 29:*420–425, 1974.
37. Baker M, Dorzab RJ, Winokur G et al: Depressive disease: Classification and clinical characteristics. *Compr. Psychiatry 12:*354–365, 1971.
38. Robins E, Guze SB: Classification of affective disorders: The primary-secondary, the endogenous-reactive, and the neurotic-psychotic concepts. In: Williams TA, Katz MM, Shield JA (eds) *Recent Advances in the Psychobiology of the Depressive Illnesses* Washington, DC, U.S. Government Printing Office, 1972.
39. Feighner JP, Robins E, Guze SB et al.: Diagnostic criteria for use in psychiatric research. *Arch. Gen. Psychiatry 26:*57–63, 1972.
40. Winokur G: The types of affective disorders. *J. Nerv. Ment. Dis. 156:*82–96, 1973.
41. Schildkraut JJ, Klein DF: The classification and treatment of depressive disorders. In: Shader RI (ed) *Manual of Psychiatric Therapeutics.* Boston, Little, Brown, 1975.
42. Klein DF: Endogenomorphic depression. *Arch. Gen. Psychiatry 31:*447–454, 1974.
43. Schildkraut JJ: *Neuropsychopharmacology and the Affective Disorders.* Boston, Little, Brown, 1970.
44. Rosenthal SH: Involutional depression. In: Arieti S, Brody SB (eds) *American Handbook of Psychiatry* (2nd ed.). New York, Basic Books, 1974.
45. Schildkraut JJ: Norepinephrine metabolites as biochemical criteria for classifying depressive disorders and predicting responses to treatment: Preliminary findings. *Am. J. Psychiatry 130:*695–699, 1973.
46. Beckmann H, Goodwin FK: Antidepressant response to tricyclics and urinary MHPG in unipolar patients. *Arch. Gen. Psychiatry 32:*17–21, 1975.
47. Maas JW, Fawcett JA, Dekirmenjian H: Catecholamine metabolism, depressive illness, and drug response. *Arch Gen. Psychiatry 26:*252–262, 1972.
48. Maas JW: Biogenic amines and depression: Biochemical and pharmacological separation of two types of depression. *Arch. Gen. Psychiatry 32:*1357–1361, 1975.

2

The Biology of Affective Illness: Amine Neurotransmitters and Drug Response

FREDERICK K. GOODWIN and WILLIAM Z. POTTER

For years psychiatrists have speculated that the depressive syndrome, especially in its more severe forms, reflects a biological dysfunction at some level. This chapter will review certain biological and pharmacological approaches toward understanding affective illnesses and choosing specific treatments for them. The belief that biology is somehow involved in the syndrome of depression has its roots in a number of important observations, some of which are presented in depth elsewhere in this volume. Genetic studies suggest that individuals inherit a predisposition toward the depressive syndrome.[1,2] Careful comparative studies of pharmacotherapy with and without psychotherapy consistently demonstrate the effectiveness of antidepressant drugs; it is this fact, above all others, which points to an involvement of biology in depression. Two other features of major depressions suggesting a biological contribution are their predictable duration and high probability of recurrence. Recent long-term studies from Europe indicate that the majority of major depressive and affective illnesses are recurrent.[3,4] From 55% to 85% of affective illnesses requiring extensive medical intervention or hospitalization are found to be recurrent when patients are followed over time.[3,4] This holds true whether the diagnosis is depression (unipolar) or manic-depressive illness (bipolar).

FREDERICK K. GOODWIN and WILLIAM Z. POTTER • Clinical Psychobiology Branch, National Institute of Mental Health, Bethesda, Maryland.

THE SPECTRUM OF DEPRESSION

The issues of biology and classification are dealt with comprehensively in another chapter. For our purposes here it is useful to consider briefly a model for conceptualizing biological factors in affective illness (see Figure 1). As a general rule, the closer the depressed patient is to the right end of the spectrum, the more likely he is to have a biological dysfunction which may respond to pharmacotherapy. In this model there is no definite cutoff point for defining *biological* depression and there is a large intermediate area of the spectrum in which biological *and* environmental factors may be operative. Moreover, the features at either end of the spectrum are not mutually exclusive.[5] A more complete discussion of this model can be found elsewhere.[6]

Factor-analytic studies make it clear that the distinction between "reactive" (or neurotic) and "endogenous" depression rests on the presence or absence of endogenous features, not the presence or absence of neurotic symptoms or reactive features.[7,8] In other words, some patients with the endogenous syndrome may have neurotic or reactive features (including clear precipitating events)[9,10] while some may not.

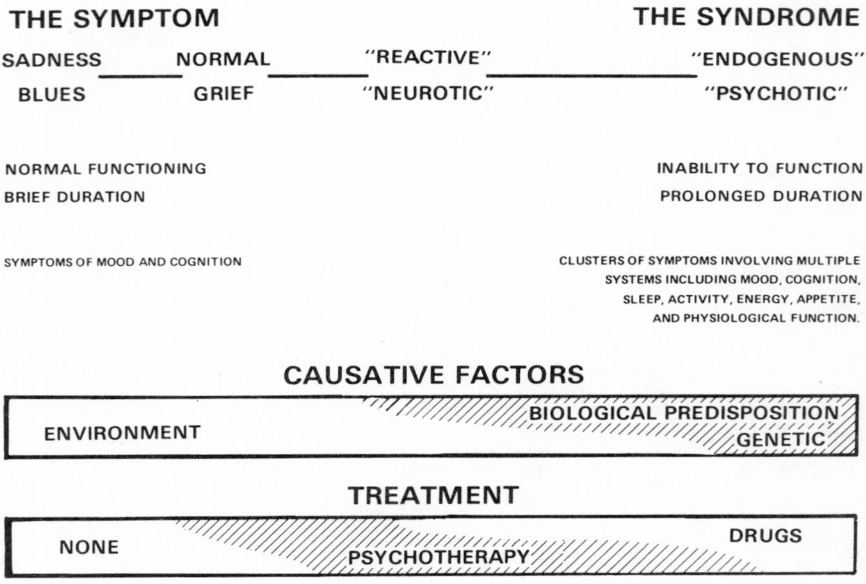

THE SYMPTOM — THE SYNDROME

SADNESS / BLUES — NORMAL / GRIEF — "REACTIVE" / "NEUROTIC" — "ENDOGENOUS" / "PSYCHOTIC"

NORMAL FUNCTIONING
BRIEF DURATION

INABILITY TO FUNCTION
PROLONGED DURATION

SYMPTOMS OF MOOD AND COGNITION

CLUSTERS OF SYMPTOMS INVOLVING MULTIPLE SYSTEMS INCLUDING MOOD, COGNITION, SLEEP, ACTIVITY, ENERGY, APPETITE, AND PHYSIOLOGICAL FUNCTION.

CAUSATIVE FACTORS

ENVIRONMENT — BIOLOGICAL PREDISPOSITION — GENETIC

TREATMENT

NONE — PSYCHOTHERAPY — DRUGS

Figure 1. Depression—a spectrum.

On the other hand, the diagnosis of neurotic or reactive depression depends on the relative absence of endogenous features. Confusion in the use of these dichotomous terms (particularly *reactive* vs. *endogenous* and *neurotic* vs. *psychotic*) could, for instance, lead to the withholding of medication in depression because neurotic symptoms were present. The issue of severity also needs clarification. It is obvious that the overall severity of the problem generally increases toward the endogenous end of the spectrum. Nevertheless, it is possible for an individual with a severe neurotic depression (absence of endogenous features) to be in more distress than another patient with a mild or moderate depression having endogenous features. Therefore, to think about depression as either psychological or biological (reactive *or* endogenous) is misleading. The model of depression as a spectrum provides a framework for investigating multiple etiologies.

THE AMINE HYPOTHESES OF AFFECTIVE DISORDER

The discovery of effective drug treatments for affective illness (depression and mania) stimulated the neuropharmacological investigations which have provided a scientific basis for current hypotheses on the pathophysiology of affective disorder. The bulk of this work has focused on dopamine and norepinephrine, the two neurotransmitter catecholamines, and on the indoleamine, serotonin. These amines appear to function as neurotransmitters in critical integrative pathways in the central nervous system. Over the past fifteen years, basic research has identified and categorized the amine neuronal systems as primary regulatory circuits in those areas of the brain which subserve functions broadly related to appetitive behaviors, drives, arousal, "emotions" (including their neuroendocrine and psychophysiological concomitants) and to the integration of these functions with a wide range of other brain components. The neuroanatomical distribution of these neurons as we currently understand them may be briefly described. The cell bodies of amine neurons are primarily located toward the midline in the upper brain stem and midbrain, with very long axonal projections going throughout the limbic system, cerebral cortex, neocortex, hypothalamus, and lower brain stem. This distribution provides interaction with the major functional areas of the brain.[11,12] Estimates have been made that a single nerve cell body receiving input from multiple sources can synapse with as many as 75,000 neurons.[12] Thus, a relatively small number of neurons can have relatively great functional significance.

Our understanding of the monoamine neurons and some of their functional roles explains why those interested in the pathophysiology of affective illness and the mechanisms of action of antidepressant and antimanic drugs have focused on these three neurotransmitters. It seems unlikely that the biological substrate of a syndrome as complex as affective illness, with its interrelated cognitive, emotional, psychomotor, appetitive, and autonomic manifestations, would be found in highly localized, specialized systems. Instead one looks for systems that are complex, widely distributed throughout the brain, and essentially integrative in function. The monoamine systems meet these qualifications.

A short review of our evolving knowledge of amine function in the central nervous system is helpful when discussing current biological hypotheses related to affective illness. Using norepinephrine as a model, Figure 2A schematically illustrates amine function at a nerve ending.

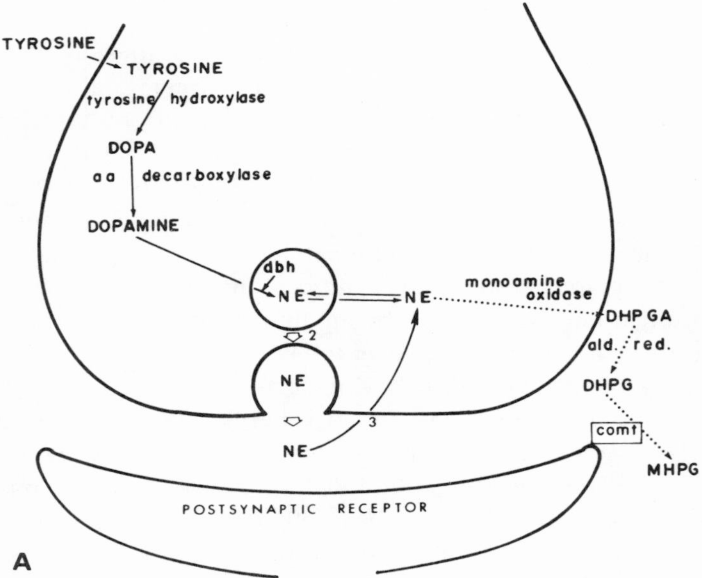

Figure 2. Monoaminergic synapses—proposed schema. 1 = active amino acid uptake; 2 = migration and exocytotic release of transmitter into synaptic cleft; 3 = active reuptake of transmitter, a process blocked by tricyclic antidepressants. In this simplified model the association of monoamine oxidase with mitochondria in the nerve terminal is not shown. (A) *Noradrenergic*. Symbols: aa = amino acid; dbh = dopamine-beta-hydroxylase; NE = norepinephrine; DHPGA = dihydroxyphenylglyceraldehyde; ald. red. = aldehyde reductase; DHPG = dihydroxyphenylglycol; comt = catechol-*O*-methyltransferase (associated

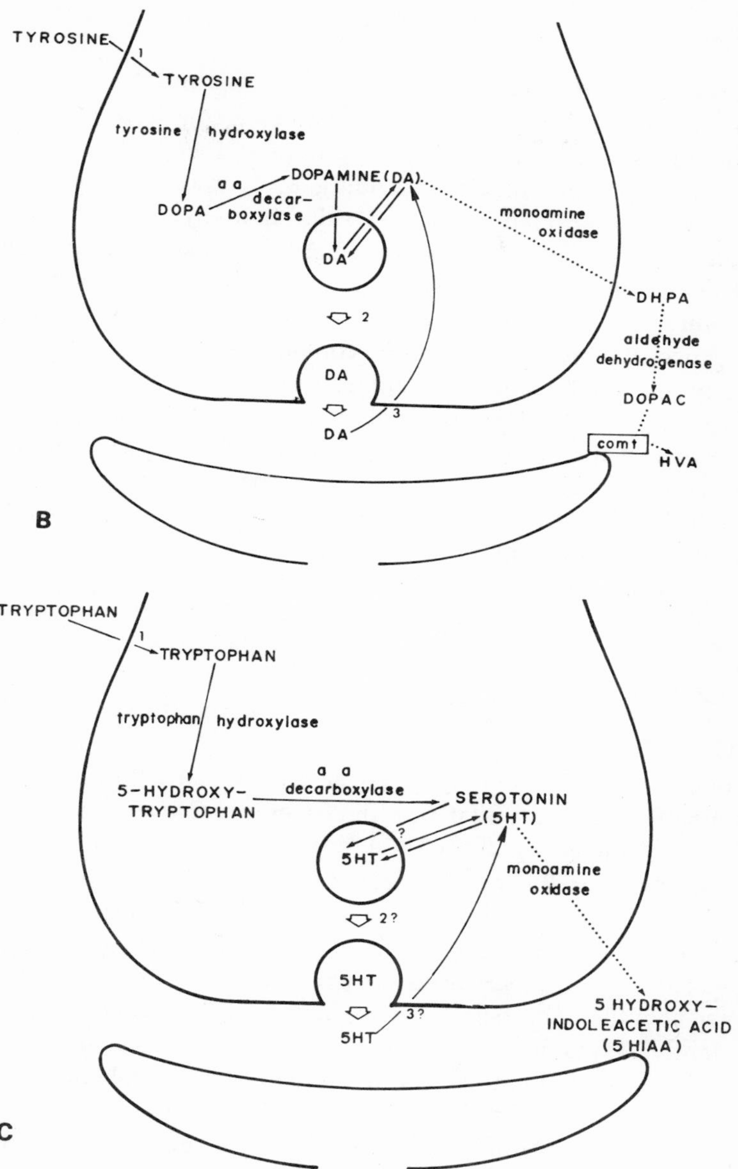

with the postsynaptic receptor membrane); MHPG = 3-methoxy-4-hydroxyphenylglycol. (B) *Dopaminergic.* Abbreviations the same except DHPA = dihydroxyphenylaldehyde; DOPAC = dihydroxyphenylacetic acid; HVA = homovanillic acid. (C) *Serotonergic.* "?" indicates absence of clear data but assumption that process is similar to noradrenergic. The conversion of 5HT to 5HIAA requires an additional oxidation by aldehyde dehydrogenase, which is omitted since no intermediate product is detected.

First, tyrosine, a dietary amino acid, is taken up into the neuron by an active transport process where it undergoes a ring hydroxylation (the rate-limiting step in norepinephrine synthesis), followed by a decarboxylation to dopamine, and then undergoes a process of uptake into a storage vesicle with an associated side chain hydroxylation to form norepinephrine. With the arrival of a nerve impulse, a complex process is set in motion involving calcium and other ionic shifts. As a result of these shifts, the vesicle migrates to the inner wall of the neuronal membrane, fuses with it, and releases its contents into the synaptic junction. There the neurotransmitter can interact with the postsynaptic receptor to set in motion another neuronal event. An active transport process takes some of the released neurotransmitter back into the neuron for restorage or metabolism by monoamine oxidase. Pathways for the synthesis of dopamine and serotonin are also illustrated in Figures 2B and 2C. Detailed discussions of amine function at nerve endings and synthetic pathways are available elsewhere.[13,14]

The initial suggestion of a relationship between the functional state of these neurotransmitters and the clinical state of depression was the result of a chance observation concerning side effects of the drug reserpine. The widespread use of this drug in the early 1950s as an antihypertensive agent also caused a significant number of patients to experience symptoms of depression.[15,16,17] At about the same time it was found in animal experiments that reserpine was capable of depleting nerve endings of their stores of serotonin, dopamine, and norepinephrine.[18,19]

Shortly after the observations concerning reserpine, there came another serendipitous observation that the use of a drug for a medical condition could have effects on mood. Some patients being treated with iproniazid for their tuberculosis were noted to have mood elevation with a reversal of the depression often associated with chronic illness.[20] Concomitantly, it was independently discovered that this drug was capable of elevating brain amine levels by inhibiting the metabolizing enzyme monoamine oxidase (MAO) (Figures 2A–C).[21] It was shown in animals that a series of MAO inhibitors could prevent or reverse the syndrome of sedation and depression produced by reserpine.[22] Thus, one had the observation of a mood-elevating drug (MAO inhibitor) that also elevated brain amines and a mood-depressing drug (reserpine) that decreased brain amines. These observations became the twin cornerstones of the amine hypothesis.[23,24,25] One of the original formulators of the hypothesis, Dr. Schildkraut,[25] presents current refinements elsewhere in this volume. (See Chapter 3.)

In its simplest form, the amine hypothesis states that depression is associated with a functional deficit of one or more brain neurotransmitter amines at specific central synapses; conversely, mania is associated with a functional excess of one or more of these amines.[25] Later it was demonstrated that the tricyclic compounds with antidepressant properties[26] blocked presynaptic amine reuptake and thereby increased the availability of amines at receptor sites.[27,28] Conversely, lithium, an effective antimanic agent,[29] was found to enhance reuptake[30] and to inhibit release[31] of amines, actions which presumably decrease functionally active transmitters at the receptor—an effect "opposite" to the tricyclic antidepressants. Because the tricyclic antidepressants have only a weak effect on the uptake of dopamine compared to their effect on serotonin and norepinephrine (reviewed in reference 32), the amine hypothesis has focused on these latter two amines.

A variety of difficulties (such as species variation, differences in the time frame of clinical effects vs. neurochemical effects in animals, and lack of an acceptable animal model for depression) serves to limit the interpretation of these "pharmacological bridges." In addition, there are some clinical observations which do not easily fit into the hypothesis that depression is associated with a functional deficit in central amines, while mania is associated with a functional excess. First, drugs that are stimulants in normal individuals (e.g., cocaine, amphetamine) and which increase amine function at the nerve synapse are not generally found to be therapeutic in patients suffering a major depression.[33,34] Conversely, drugs that do have antidepressant activity are not stimulants in normals.[35] Second, there are two new drugs with antidepressant properties, iprindole[36] and mianserin,[37] which have no apparent effect on amines at the synapse.[36,38] A third inconsistency relates to the clinical efficacy of the MAO inhibitors, which apparently have a spectrum of effectiveness different from that of the tricyclic antidepressants. This is difficult to reconcile with a conclusion implicit in the amine hypothesis, namely that both types of antidepressants work by increasing brain amine function (Table I).

In addition, there are problems with the interpretations of the clinical effects of those drugs which formed the foundations of the catecholamine hypothesis. In relation to the original reserpine observations, it should be noted that the incidence of patients experiencing major depressive symptoms (i.e., those analogous to endogenous depression) was almost identical to the incidence of individuals with prior histories of depression.[39] Thus it appears more likely that reserpine is

Table I. Drug Amine Relationships

Drug	Effect on amines at receptor	Behavioral effects in man: Normals	Predisposed to affective illness	Depressed patients	Manic patients
MAOI	↑	No effect or mild sedation	Can precipitate mania	Some antidepressant activity	?
Tricyclics	↑	No effect or mild sedation	Can precipitate mania Prevents recurrences of depression (?)	Antidepressant	Antimanic (?)
Amphetamine	↑	Stimulation	Can precipitate mania (?)	Poor antidepressant	Antimanic (?)
Cocaine	↑	Stimulation	Can precipitate mania (?)	Poor antidepressant	?
L-DOPA	↑ (DA,NE)	No effect	Can precipitate hypomania	Activation without antidepressant effect	?
L-Tryptophan	↑ (5HT)	Sedation	?	Antidepressant (?)	Antimanic (?)
L-5HTP	↑ (5HT)	?	Prevents recurrences of mania and depression (?)	Antidepressant (?)	?
Reserpine	↓	Sedation	Can precipitate depression	?	Sedation and/or tranquilization
Lithium	↓	No effect or mild sedation	Prevents recurrences of mania and depression	Moderate antidepressant effect in some	Antimanic
AMPT	↓ (DA,NE)	Sedation	?	Sedation	Antimanic (?)
Fusaric acid (DBH inhibitor)	↓ (NE)	No effect	?	No effect	Not antimanic—psychosis increased
PCPA	↓ (5HT)	↑ Anxiety	?	No specific effect	?
Iprindole	None	?	?	Antidepressant	?
Mianserin	None	?	?	Antidepressant	?

capable of precipitating depression in susceptible individuals rather than of inducing it *de novo*, an important distinction. Additionally, lithium has antidepressant effects in some patients, both acutely and prophylactically; this finding is difficult to reconcile with its ability to decrease functional amines, which of course *is* consistent with its antimanic effects. Many of these findings (see Table I) are reviewed in greater detail elsewhere.[40] It should be clear that given the discrepancies between theory, animal studies, and clinical observations there must follow efforts to evaluate amine function directly in patients.

STUDIES OF AMINE METABOLITES IN AFFECTIVE DISORDER

In the preceding section we discussed the basic amine hypothesis of affective disorders and some of the problems with that hypothesis. The clinical studies stimulated by the amine hypothesis have been performed and continue to be performed in diverse settings, so that methodologies are not coordinated. This observation is necessary because in this section the presentation of findings may initially appear to be a list of contradictory statements. Since amine function in humans is being actively studied and debated, it is unreasonable to disregard any relevant reports. However, it is not possible to provide a comprehensive explanation for the findings. Therefore, in this section we will describe the common methodological ground that does exist, summarize relevant findings from the last eight years, and discuss whether general conclusions are possible. The next section will be concerned with specific areas in which coordinated studies of amine function may be clinically useful.

The common methodological ground involves the study of amine *metabolites* in man rather than the measurements of unmetabolized dopamine, norepinephrine, or serotonin. Aside from the technical difficulties inherent in measuring unmetabolized amines in blood, urine, or cerebrospinal fluid (CSF), fluctuations are so great that differences between groups have been virtually impossible to find. In the urine, a metabolite measure can give an index of total output over a period of time, i.e., an integrated measure. CSF metabolites, although less fluctuant than blood levels, are not truly integrated measures.

Five-hydroxy-indoleacetic acid (5HIAA) is the major metabolite of serotonin, both centrally and peripherally.[41] It has generally been assumed that brain serotonin metabolism cannot be studied in the urine because of the large peripheral contribution to urinary 5HIAA. Although a recent study has called this assumption into question,[42] only CSF measurements of 5HIAA are relied upon at this time. Dopamine is metabolized principally to 3-methoxy-4-hydroxyphenylacetic acid (HVA) and to a lesser extent to 3,4-dihydroxyphenylacetic acid (DOPAC).[43] The question of what proportion of urinary dopamine metabolites originate in the brain is unsettled; in Parkinsonism, where dopamine deficiency is known to exist centrally, urinary HVA has been reported both as unchanged and as decreased.[44–47] Until further information is available, one must remain cautious about the use of urinary HVA as a reflection of brain dopamine metabolism in man.

On the other hand, studies of norepinephrine metabolites in the urine offer considerable promise. The major metabolites of norepinephrine in the urine are 3-methoxy-4-hydroxymandelic acid (VMA) and 3-methoxy-4-hydroxyphenylglycol (MHPG).[48] Enzyme studies in animal species indicate that aldehyde reductase predominates over aldehyde dehydrogenase in the brain, whereas the opposite is true in peripheral tissues.[49] This suggests that the aldehydes of norepinephrine follow a predominantly reductive pathway (to MHPG) in the central nervous system and an oxidative pathway (to VMA) in peripheral tissues. Although the urinary amine itself is predominantly of peripheral origin, studies in different species suggest that from 25% to 60% of the urinary MHPG has its origins in the metabolism of norepinephrine in the brain.[50,51] Recent work[52] utilizing [^{14}C]dopamine infusions suggests that the majority of urinary MHPG in man has its origins in brain pools of norepinephrine, while virtually all of the urinary VMA results from metabolism of peripheral norepinephrine. Consequently, given the questionable central origins of other urinary amine metabolites, clinical studies have focused on MHPG. This metabolite has been reported to be low in "endogenous" depression compared to its level in controls,[53] to increase after recovery from depression,[54] and to be higher in the manic phase than in the depressed phase of bipolar affective illness.[54–58] Other studies of urinary MHPG concentration will be presented later in the chapter where more specific applications of amine metabolite data are considered.

In contrast to the rather limited results of urinary studies, reports of CSF investigations have provided the major source of information of brain metabolism of amines in man. The major metabolite of dopamine in the CSF is homovanillic acid (HVA or 3-methoxy-4-hydroxyphenylacetic acid) although very low concentrations of dopamine's minor metabolite (DOPAC) have been detected.[59,60] As previously discussed, there is clear evidence for serotonin and norepinephrine that their respective major metabolites in the CSF are 5HIAA and MHPG.[40,50,51,52]

The CSF does not necessarily contain all of the amine metabolites which originate in brain tissue. It has been demonstrated by a variety of techniques, however, that changes in amine metabolism in the brain are reliably reflected in parallel changes in CSF metabolites (reviewed in reference 61). A more important methodological question in the interpretation of human CSF data concerns the extent to which the lumbar CSF reflects the ventricular CSF; various studies support the conclusion that a substantial portion of the lumbar 5HIAA and MHPG comes from the spinal cord while most, if not all, of the lumbar HVA comes from the brain (see reference 61). Even if it were to be shown that 5HIAA and MHPG in lumbar CSF mainly reflect spinal cord metabolism, these substances may still prove clinically and biologically important since many of the serotonin and norepinephrine terminals in the spinal cord originate in cell bodies localized in brainstem nuclei.

A further refinement of the CSF approach to the study of amine metabolism involves the probenecid technique. Probenecid inhibits the system which transports 5HIAA and HVA out of the CSF[62] but not the system which transports MHPG.[63] Thus, in an individual pretreated with probenecid relatively large amounts of 5HIAA and HVA accumulate in CSF and, particularly in the case of 5HIAA, probably make lumbar CSF more representative of ventricular CSF. Earlier studies in which lower doses of probenecid were used showed considerable variation in amine metabolite accumulation as a function of probenecid concentration;[64,65,66] recent studies using high (100 mg/kg) doses of probenecid reveal a modest correlation between probenecid level and metabolite accumulation.[67,68] Some groups report data from CSF obtained with and without probenecid—the term *baseline* will be used to refer to these values of CSF amines obtained from individuals not pretreated with probenecid.

An actual tabulation of amine concentrations found in the CSF of patients with affective illness reveals somewhat conflicting results. In Tables IIA and B data from both baseline and probenecid studies are presented for each of the three major neurotransmitter metabolites. Figures from the baseline and probenecid studies do not contradict each other when the general trend is reviewed. Nevertheless, we cannot

TABLE IIA. CEREBROSPINAL FLUID AMINE METABOLITES IN AFFECTIVE ILLNESS[a]

	Control		Depression		Mania	
Study	*N*	Mean S.D.	*N*	Mean S.D.	*N*	Mean S.D.
			CSF 5HIAA (ng/ml)			
Ashcroft	21	19.1 ± 4.4	24	11.1 ± 3.9	4	18.7 ± 5.4
Dencker	34	30 (median)	14	10 (median)	6	10 (median)
Fotherby	11	11.5 ± 4.1	11	12.2 ± 8.2		
			6	16.6 ± 9.4		
Coppen	20	42.3 ± 14	31	19.8 ± 8.5	18	19.7 ± 6.8
Roos	26	29 ± 7	17	31 ± 8	19	36 ± 9
Bowers	18	43.5 ± 16.8	8	34.0 ± 11.5	8	42.0 ± 10.3
van Praag	11	40 ± 24	14	17 ± 17		
Papeschi	10	28 ± 3	12	22 ± 2		
McLeod	12	32.6 ± 11.4	25	20.5 ± 12.1		
Goodwin	29	27.3 ± 1.6	85	25.5 ± 1.3	40	28.7 ± 2.5
Asberg			68	20.4 ± 7.8		
			CSF HVA (ng/ml)			
Roos	7	44 ± 31	6	29 ± 7	7	41 ± 23
Roos	39	34 ± 3	37	34 ± 4	42	59 ± 6
Bowers			8	22.7 ± 14.1	7	22.2 ± 16.3
Papeschi	18	50 ± 6	17	19 ± 4		
van Praag	12	42 ± 16	20	39 ± 16		
Goodwin and Post	28	22.4 ± 2.4	80	15.2 ± 2.1	40	25.7 ± 4.3
Subrahmanyan	12	42.4 ± 3.8	24	38.4 ± 3.4		
			MHPG (ng/ml)			
Wilk	24	16 ± 4.2	8	17.6 ± 1.2	11	31.6 ± 5.8
Post	44	15.1 ± 3.6	55	10.2 ± 2.4	26	15.4 ± 5.5
Shaw	13	10.8 ± 2.8	22	11.9 ± 2.6		
Subrahmanyan	12	21.4 ± 3.2	24	14.2 ± 2.6		

[a]Table IIa taken from Goodwin et al.[61] where individual studies are referenced, except for Subrahmanyan[69] and Asberg[70] results added to the table.

make specific conclusions on the basis of these data. First, there is the striking variability in the data. Second, the data do not support a single amine theory of illness. Third, an analysis of the actual reports reveals a paucity of *normal* controls for CSF measurements. Fourth, there are major diagnostic uncertainties due to the heterogeneity of patients with affective illness.

More specifically, there are problems involving each amine metabolite. With regard to the norepinephrine metabolite MHPG, not only do results differ among researchers but also there are inconsistencies in

TABLE IIB. 5HIAA AND HVA FOLLOWING PROBENECID IN DEPRESSED PATIENTS[a]

	Accumulations in depressed patients as percent of controls			
	5HIAA	*N*	HVA	*N*
Sjostrom and Roos, 1972	41%[b]	(24)	40%[b]	(10)
Bowers, 1974	109%	(11)	138%	(10)
Goodwin, Post et al., 1973	78%	(6)[c]	47%[b]	(6)[c]
van Praag and Korf, 1973	69%[b]	(28)	75%[b]	(28)
Sjostrom, 1974	low[b]	(22)	low[b]	(22)

[a]Table IIB taken from Goodwin et al.[61] where individual studies are referenced.
[b]Significant, $p < .05$.
[c]Only the depressed patients studied under conditions identical to that of the controls are included. The total number of depressed patients studied with probenecid is 54.

urinary and CSF data from the same group.[71] This phenomenon will be recalled in the discussion of subgroups. In the case of serotonin, none of the CSF studies of its metabolite, 5HIAA, are consistent with a "too little (in depression)—too much (in mania)" model,[72] but much of the data could support a version of the "serotonin hypothesis" which postulates a serotonin abnormality underlying *both* mania and depression.[73] Finally, with regard to dopamine, some of the HVA data might support a hypothesis of a dopamine deficiency in depression. Yet the results in mania are confused by higher baseline levels in certain studies (perhaps secondary to activity differences) compared to low accumulations following probenecid.

Even though a general conclusion is elusive, the overall direction of the evidence is for an *average* decrease in all three amine metabolites; this requires some explanation. One possibility would be a single abnormality that affects all amine systems. An alternative view might postulate subgroups in which a given amine abnormality predominates, with each subgroup representing a portion of the overall population and accounting for the low average for the whole. It is to this second possibility that we will now address our attention.

APPROACHES TO SUBGROUPS IN THE AFFECTIVE DISORDERS

It is apparent that on the basis of current knowledge a simple theory of amine deficit or excess in affective illness cannot be substantiated. 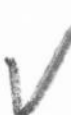

Given a diagnostically homogeneous population (i.e., patients with major primary affective illness), can biochemical and pharmacological measures be used to help identify and differentiate subpopulations? Figure 3 illustrates a model which provides a useful framework for putting biological and pharmacological factors into the perspective of interrelationships between three available spheres of information about a patient. Whatever the sphere of information—clinical presentation, biological findings, or pharmacological response—one may determine for any single variable its distribution in the population; that is, is it distributed normally or bimodally, or is it clustered in some other way? If the distribution were nonrandom and nonnormal (particularly if it were clearly bimodal), the likelihood of meaningful subgroups would be enhanced. However, the pattern of distribution of any single variable is not sufficient to identify or to rule out a meaningful subgroup. The important issue is how the variance in one set of data might be understood in relation to the variance in other sets of data from the same population. Elsewhere in this volume Dr. Schildkraut and his associates propose a discrimination equation to generate D-type ("depression-type") scores. Their work is an example of using several variables, obtained by measuring urinary concentrations of catecholamine metabolites, to identify meaningful subgroups. They also address the possibility of using biological data to predict pharmacological response, thus providing subgrouping within a second sphere. (See Chapter 3.)

Note that there are six numbered arrows in the model illustrated in Figure 3; each represents a different approach to the subgroup question. The following are examples of six paired questions (real or hypothetical)

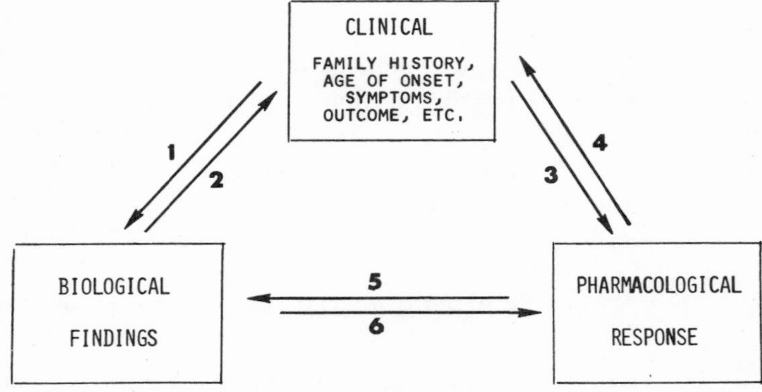

Figure 3. Spheres of information applied to the identification of subgroups.

whose numbers correspond to the individual arrows as numbered in the figure:

1. Are unipolar and bipolar depressed patients different in regard to urinary MHPG execretion?
2. Are differences in urinary MHPG execretion among patients with affective illness reflected in different clinical profiles?
3. Do unipolar and bipolar depressed patients respond differently to lithium?
4. Does lithium responsiveness correspond to a clinically definable subgroup of affective illness?
5. Are differential responses to specific types of tricyclic antidepressants associated with different urinary MHPG concentrations?
6. Does a bimodal distribution of urinary MHPG concentration in depressed patients predict differential response to antidepressants?

In order to answer these questions and to confirm the existence of a proposed subgroup, one needs consistent data from the clinical, biological, and pharmacological spheres. Probably the major difficulty for those seeking to establish subgroups through correlations between these spheres lies in the many potential sources of variance present in any set of data. In this field, the most fundamental question concerning variance relates to clinical diagnosis, an area addressed in detail elsewhere in this volume.

Before we can consider whether investigations of biological and pharmacological factors can contribute to more precise and meaningful diagnoses, we must consider the multiple sources of variance in these areas. In exploring variance in biological data, we consider whether a given source of variance is likely to be *intrinsic* to the pathophysiology of the illness and therefore likely to be useful in differentiating subgroups, or *incidental* and therefore a potential artifact. As an illustration of this point, Table III lists various factors which have been reported to affect the level of amine metabolites in at least one clinical study. Note that only a few of the factors can be designated as specific or nonspecific; most of them represent a complicated picture in which a given source of variance may or may nor contribute to the illness itself. Rather than discuss each point in detail, we will selectively illustrate the complexities involved in attempting to evaluate or control for any of these variables in biological studies of psychiatric patients. Consider, for example, age

TABLE III. HETEROGENEITY IN BIOLOGICAL STUDIES OF PSYCHIATRIC ILLNESS: SOME CONTRIBUTING CLINICAL FACTORS

Factors not likely to be specific to the illness or subgroup (no primary etiologic relationship)
Age distribution
Sex distribution
Phase of illness studied
Factors which may or may not be specific to the illness or subgroup
Physiological differences (blood pressure, temperature, renal clearance, etc.)
Activity
Diet
Clinical state differences (anxiety, agitation, retardation, psychosis, etc.)
Time of day studied (diurnal variation)
Time of year studied (annual rhythms)
Factors likely to be specific to the illness or subgroup
Genetic differences (family history)
Age of onset
State-independent clinical differences (e.g., history of mania)

distribution: if a relationship between age and the biological variable is independent of the subgroups under question, its contribution to the variance can be eliminated from the data by an analysis of covariance. Thus, we found essentially the same modest but significant correlation between urinary MHPG and age in both our unipolar and bipolar depressed patients.[74] In this instance, removing the contribution of age resulted in increasing the significance of the unipolar–bipolar differences in MHPG (see the section below).

Differences in sex distribution within study groups can also contribute to significant amine metabolite differences. For example, females have significantly higher probenecid-induced accumulations of 5HIAA and HVA than do males in our affectively ill population. For urinary MHPG, the sex differences are in the opposite direction, males having levels 20–30% higher than females[74,75]; a similar trend is seen in our CSF MHPG data. Differences of this magnitude require either standardization of sex distribution among comparison populations or else separate analyses of group differences for males and females.

A particularly critical issue in the interpretation of biological data in affective disorders involves the *phase of the illness* in which the data is obtained. It would be ideal to study a patient longitudinally throughout the illness—that is, during the early acute phase, during the stable and waning phases, and following recovery. Considerations of the phase of the illness are particularly relevant to the study of subgroups in affective illness because the phenomenon of *cyclicity* may be variably expressed in a population. For example, in the bipolar subgroup and in some unipolar patients the inherent cyclicity is particularly striking. Cyclicity implies that what might otherwise be termed *remissions* and *relapses* are simply part of the disease process. Most metabolite studies have not attempted to control for the stage of illness (e.g., early vs. late depression).

Note that in Table III diet and physical activity are included among those factors which may or may not be specific to the illness or subgroups. Why? Recently we have noted clear differences between hospitalized bipolar depressed patients and normal controls in urinary MHPG responses to changes in diet and activity. In the patients, discontinuation of a low monoamine diet resulted in significant increases in urinary MHPG (averaging 70% for the group), while this dietary alteration in normal controls studied under identical conditions on the same ward produced no change. Similarly, moderate exercise produced substantial increases in MHPG in bipolar depressed patients but had no effect in normal controls.[58] The possibility of a unipolar–bipolar difference in this response has not yet been evaluated. There are important implications of these results. First, normals are not suitable subjects in whom to evaluate the contribution of some factors to amine metabolite variance in patients. Second, within a population of patients these factors may themselves differentiate subgroups of affective illness. We have discussed only some of the sources of variance listed in Table III. No amine metabolite studies have controlled for all these sources of variance. In no study of depression has the phase of the illness been adequately documented. For some variables (such as anxiety, agitation, and psychomotor retardation), adequate methods for reliable quantification have been lacking. Some of the conflicting findings which we have reviewed may be resolved as we become more able to account for such variables.

As noted by other authors in this volume, pharmacological studies must also be interpreted with caution. There is considerable interest in examining the relationships between drug response and pretreatment clinical or biological variables, especially the latter. Just as was discussed above in regard to biological data, there are incidental sources of variance in drug response which must be considered before differences in drug response are cited as evidence of biochemical subgroups. It is not our purpose to review this extensive and complex area but rather to highlight some of the key issues (outlined in Table IV). We wish to

TABLE IV. SOME PROBLEMS IN THE EVALUATION OF DIFFERENTIAL DRUG RESPONSE

1. Non-drug-related factors contributing to improvement (hospitalization, psychotherapy, "spontaneous" change)
2. Drug-related factors, but not limited to the specific drug under evaluation (IMI vs. AMI?)
3. Differential drug compliance
4. Differential threshold for side effects
5. Variability in drug metabolism and blood levels
6. Differences in ratio of active metabolites with differential amine effects
7. Biochemical heterogeneity in the depressed population

distinguish these issues from ordinary errors in experimental design (such as not randomizing assignment to pretreatment groups) and analytical limitations (such as imprecise quantitation of substances—see reference 71). An example of a problem listed in Table IV is one concerning the issue of hospitalization: it is estimated that among patients hospitalized for depression up to 25% will improve substantially within the first week due to the effects of the hospitalization alone.[76] Thus, if a drug trial is initiated immediately upon admission, the response group will be contaminated with "false positives," distorting any possible biological differences between responders and nonresponders.

A major pharmacological problem involves factors which affect the amount of active drug reaching the brain in an individual patient. Two of these factors are differences in drug compliance (especially in outpatient studies) and differences in threshold for side effects. For example, a nonresponder who has skipped doses or could not get beyond a low dose because of exaggerated sensitivity to side effects may be a good "false negative" and therefore obscure possible drug response–biological relationships. A more fundamental problem concerning the amount of active drug getting to the brain stems from wide interpatient variability in the metabolism of drugs, particularly the tricyclic antidepressants. This variability in metabolism results, of course, in comparable variation in blood and tissue concentrations of drugs.[77] Thus, in a trial where standardized doses are given, some patients who fail to respond may really be "false negatives" because they never achieve an adequate blood level of the drug. A recent study in which concentrations of tricyclic antidepressants were measured in an outpatient population showed a dramatic variation in actual concentrations encountered in practice.[78] In patients prescribed the same dose of imipramine (200 mg/day) the plasma concentration of imipramine plus its active metabolite desmethylimipramine varied from 20 ng/ml up to 800 ng/ml. Similar variation was found at other doses.[78] Moreover, it is not necessarily correct to assume that if enough antidepressant is given one has achieved therapeutic concentrations. Careful clinical investigations in Scandinavia have shown that nortriptyline is ineffective on either side of a relatively narrow plasma concentration range, and as many as 80% of nonresponders on supposed "therapeutic" doses actually have concentrations that are too high.[79,80] This finding has gained strong support from an American study showing that nortriptyline is effective only at a plasma concentration of 50 ng/ml to 140 ng/ml.[81]

Another consideration in the evaluation of responses to the tricyclic antidepressants is the interpatient variation in the ratios of active metabolites of the drugs. This source of variance can be a problem in establishing relationships between clinical response to different tricyclics and measures of brain amine metabolites since, as we will discuss below, there is evidence suggesting that different tricyclic metabolites have different effects on specific brain amine systems. These difficulties cannot be avoided until steady state blood level determinations become a part of therapeutic trials, as they already are in lithium trials.

PROPOSED RELATIONSHIPS OF BIOLOGICAL FINDINGS TO CLINICAL SUBGROUPS

The unipolar–bipolar distinction introduced by Leonhard in 1959[82] as a clinical classification of hospitalized depressed patients continues to gain acceptance. Significant differences between unipolar and bipolar patients are found in a wide number of areas. Even though all the findings have not been replicated, there is an impressive amount of evidence from clinical, biological, and pharmacological spheres that this is a valid distinction. This issue is reviewed in more detail elsewhere.[83]

An example of the application of the unipolar–bipolar dichotomy to the exploration of clinical–biological subgroup relationships (arrow 1 in Figure 3) is its usefulness in pinpointing possible sources of disagreement among investigators. Our group was unable to replicate the results of Maas et al.,[75] who reported low urinary MHPG in patients with primary depressive illness as compared with controls. However, when the data from the unipolar and bipolar depressed patients were examined separately, the source of discrepancy was located.[74] These data are presented in Table V, along with data from a related study of Schildkraut.[84] All three investigative groups report essentially the same mean values for the bipolar patients, with the discrepancy arising in the unipolar group. This is not surprising because diagnostic agreement is more likely in bipolar patients, whose history of mania provide clinicians with an unusually clear and dramatic "marker." The unipolar diagnosis, on the other hand, tends to include a more heterogeneous group of patients. Hopefully, the use of Research Diagnostic Criteria[85] in the future will lead to the collection of sufficient numbers of more precisely diagnosed unipolar patients.

As noted earlier, clinical–biological subgroup relationships can also be approached from the other direction—as indicated by arrow 2 in Figure 3. Recently we have found an apparent bimodal distribution in cerebrospinal fluid 5HIAA (following probenecid administration) among a group of drug-free, hospitalized patients diagnosed as having primary affective disorder.[86] This finding is consistent with Asberg's Scandinavian study based on nonprobenecid spinal taps.[70] In exploring clinical features that might differentiate the two serotonin metabolite subgroups, we examined the relative distribution of unipolar and bipolar diagnoses in the two populations and found no significant difference. However, sex distribution was different in the two metabolite groups, with an overrepresentation of females in the high-5HIAA group; reanalysis of Asberg's data has identified the same sex distribution difference.[87]

Although low- and high-5HIAA subgroups have been defined experimentally, corresponding clinical subgroups have not been clearly characterized. Our findings of an apparent bimodal distribution of cerebrospinal fluid 5HIAA included both unipolar and bipolar depressed patients; in the report by the Scandinavian group, the unipolar–bipolar distinction was not discussed. A further report from the Scandinavian group of an increased incidence of successful and attempted suicides among the low-5HIAA subgroup[88] suggests that this biological subgroup may have behavioral correlates. Careful scrutiny of the interrelationships between low 5HIAA, age of onset, sex, and polarity will be necessary to assess properly the meaning of associations between clinical, biochemical, and drug response variables.

The investigation of neuroendocrine dysfunction in the affective disorders provides a different approach to biological subgroups. Monoamine transmitters have been shown to modulate the synthesis

TABLE V. URINARY MHPG IN SUBGROUPS OF DEPRESSED PATIENTS (μg/24 HRS)

	Bipolar	Unipolar	Schizoaffective	Controls	Comments
Maas et al.[75]	916[a] (N = 5)	1070 (N = 5)	—	1348 (N = 21)	Controls were outpatients. Means for groups computed after elimination of non-P.A.D. patients.
Schildkraut et al.[84]	1240 (N = 5)	1800 (N = 6)	800 (N = 1)	—	Study reported difference between "manic-depressive depression" and "chronic characterologic depression."
Goodwin and Beckmann[74]	1020[a] (N = 11)	1623 (N = 19)	880 (N = 5)	1350 (N = 15)	

[a] Significantly lower than controls.

and release of a number of hypothalamic peptides and pituitary hormones.[89] Thus, examination of these pituitary hormones in the plasma can shed light on the functional activity of monoamine systems. Moreover, these peptides and hormones may themselves have either direct behavioral effects or influence the metabolism of monoamine or other central nervous system regulators. A recent symposium focused on current studies related to the significant interface between monoamine function and neuroendocrine secretion.[90]

Recent studies in our laboratory have attempted to examine directly monoamine–neuroendocrine relationships in affective illness. Following up earlier reports,[91] we found a significantly elevated 24-hour urinary free cortisol secretion in unipolar depressed patients compared to control subjects,[92] additionally noting a positive correlation between urinary free cortisol and cerebrospinal fluid 5HIAA. This is consistent with a variety of data which suggest that serotonin is the neurotransmitter primarily responsible for driving the hypothalamic–pituitary–adrenal axis in man.[89] In a different study, the thyroid-stimulating hormone (TSH) response to thyrotropin-releasing hormone (TRH) was shown to be significantly blunted in unipolar depressed patients compared to controls.[93] Again, among the unipolar depressed patients a significant positive correlation was noted between the probenecid-induced accumulation of 5HIAA in the CSF and the TSH response. This CSF amine metabolite correlation is consistent with the evidence that pharmacologic agents which increase functional serotonergic activity blunt the TSH response to exogenous TRH administration.[94]

In our discussion of biological–clinical subgroup relationships we have focused primarily on serotonin function and metabolism. As already mentioned, Schildkraut et al. (this volume) discuss similar issues with respect to norepinephrine and its metabolites.

PHARMACOLOGICAL RESPONSE AND POSSIBLE RELATIONSHIPS TO SUBGROUPS IN DEPRESSION

Controlled studies of pharmacological response in affective illness primarily focus on antidepressants and lithium. The psychopharmacology of depression is discussed in detail in other chapters (see Kline, Chapter 6, and Cole, Chapters 7 and 8). Investigations of the tricyclic antidepressants are particularly relevant to our discussion since basic questions about clinical and biological subgroups may be approached in terms of differential pharmacological response. Recent clinical studies have indicated that the animal data on differential amine affects of different tricyclic drugs may be applicable to the use of these drugs in patients. Specifically, in Scandinavian studies employing nortriptyline and chlorimipramine, the former produced a much greater decrease in the CSF concentration of MHPG than in that of 5HIAA, whereas chlorimipramine treatment produced a greater decrease in 5HIAA than in MHPG.[95] This is consistent with animal data suggesting that, for nortriptyline, effects on norepinephrine uptake predominate over effects on serotonin uptake, with the converse holding for chlorimipramine (Table VI). This is demonstrated in a study showing that the change of 5HIAA in the CSF is proportional to the effectiveness of chlorimipramine in the plasma in blocking serotonin uptake in brain slices.[96]

We have determined CSF concentrations of imipramine (IMI) and desmethylimipramine (DMI, the demethylated active metabolite—see Figure 4) in depressed patients treated with IMI. The concentration of DMI is greater than that of IMI in most patients, although in a few cases the ratio is reversed.[97] Decreases in cerebrospinal fluid 5HIAA during imipramine treatment are proportional to the concentration of IMI, not DMI. This finding suggests that the biological effects of IMI and DMI

TABLE VI. SUMMARY OF EFFECTS OF VARIOUS ANTIDEPRESSANT DRUGS ON BLOCKADE OF UPTAKE OF BIOGENIC AMINES[a]

Drug	Biogenic amine		
	5HT	NE	DA
Amitriptyline	++++[b]	0[c]	0
Nortriptyline	++	++	0
Imipramine	+++	++	0
Desipramine	0	++++	0

[a] Adapted from Maas.[32]
[b] Indicates most active.
[c] Indicates probable lack of activity *in vivo* at tissue levels clinically achievable.

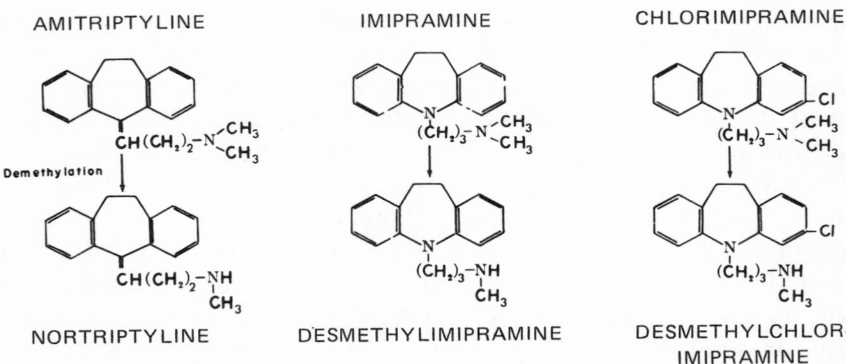

Figure 4. Major tricyclic antidepressants and their active metabolites.

may differ, and that, for most patients on imipramine, the DMI (i.e., noradrenergic) effects should predominate.

From the above we see that in cases where more than one active chemical form is present it is necessary to quantitate both accurately. Clinical studies which only report a single total concentration for the administered drug and its active metabolites are clearly difficult to interpret. One study with IMI, for example, has reported that total plasma concentrations of IMI and DMI are higher in "endogenously depressed responders" than in endogenously depressed nonresponders.[98] The same report, depending on a radioimmunoassay for quantitation, states that there is a correlation between the oral dose and the total plasma concentration of IMI plus DMI. No correlation was found between either the oral dose or plasma concentration and the amount of drug in the CSF.[98] In contrast to this report, studies using more specific mass spectrometry to quantitate IMI and DMI individually show that, while there is no correlation between oral IMI dose and its plasma concentration,[78] there is a good correlation between plasma and CSF concentration.[97]

The significance of distinguishing clearly between concentrations of DMI and IMI has more specific clinical implications. Figure 4 shows the structure of IMI, its demethylated metabolite DMI, amitriptyline (AMI), its demethylated metabolite nortriptyline (NT), and chlorimipramine and its demethylated metabolite desmethylchlorimipramine. The *in vivo* demethylation of the tricyclic antidepressants which are tertiary amines (IMI, chlorimipramine, and AMI) has important biological implications.

Several methodologies have shown that these tertiary forms of tricyclic antidepressants effectively block the uptake of serotonin into nervous tissue.[99,100] The demethylated forms (DMI, NT) have almost no effect on serotonin uptake but dramatically decrease norepinephrine uptake in similar concentrations[99,100] (Table VI).

Clinical studies show that IMI is rapidly converted to DMI, and plasma concentrations of DMI usually exceed those of IMI.[97,101] AMI is less rapidly converted to NT; thus plasma concentrations of AMI usually exceed or are equal to those of NT.[102] Table VI synthesizes these observations: AMI is more likely to have serotonergic effects (since it blocks the reuptake of serotonin), while IMI is more likely to have noradrenergic effects (since it is mainly converted to DMI, which preferentially blocks norepinephrine uptake).

These differences in drug action can assume clinical significance when we define biological subgroups of depression which respond consistently to specific drugs. Asberg, Bertilsson, Tuck et al. report that the low 5HIAA depressed subgroup does not respond to NT, whereas the high 5HIAA–low MHPG subgroup does.[103] Our finding that responders to IMI have low pretreatment 5HIAA compared to nonresponders is consistent with those Scandinavian studies (Table VII). Current studies using zimelidine, a more specific serotonin uptake inhibitor being tried in depressed patients in Sweden,[104] will help to clarify whether there is a subgroup of patients who respond only to serotonergic antidepressants.

Table VII also includes low and high urinary MHPG as predictors of antidepressant response, biological factors discussed in detail by Schildkraut et al. elsewhere in this volume. Low urinary MHPG presumably reflects decreased central norepinephrine output; thus IMI, the more noradrenergic drug, may be expected to be more effective. Conversely, higher urinary MHPG suggests that decreased central norepinephrine is *not* a significant factor; thus, AMI, a drug which has other than noradrenergic effects, may prove more effective. It is of interest that our preliminary study shows an inverse relationship between CSF 5HIAA and urinary MHPG. Twenty-four-hour urinary excretion of MHPG was analyzed in a group of 36 patients for whom data was also available on CSF 5HIAA after probenecid; MHPG excretion in the low-5HIAA group (<100 ng/ml) was significantly higher than in the high-5HIAA group ($p < .01$).[86] At this time, it is not known whether the low cerebro-

TABLE VII. AMINE METABOLITE SUBGROUPS IN DEPRESSION: SOME RELATIONSHIPS TO PHARMACOLOGICAL RESPONSE

Amine metabolite subgroups	Drug response subgroups
Low 5HIAA[a] in the CSF	Poor response to nortriptyline[79] or to imipramine[61]
Low urinary MHPG[b]	Imipramine response[75] Imipramine response in unipolars[74] Amitriptyline nonresponse[84] Amitriptyline nonresponse in unipolars[74]
Higher urinary MHPG[a]	Amitriptyline response[84] Amitriptyline response in unipolars[74] Imipramine nonresponse[75] Imipramine nonresponse in unipolars[74]

[a]5HIAA is 5-hydroxyindoleacetic acid, the major metabolite of serotonin.
[b]MHPG is 3-methoxy-4-hydroxyphenylglycol, the major metabolite of norepinephrine.

spinal fluid 5HIAA–high urinary MHPG subgroup of depressed patients consistently respond to amitriptyline, although in our data there is a trend in that direction.[87]

Biological and pharmacological response data are consistent with but not sufficient to prove the existence of two biochemically independent subgroups of depressed patients. It could be, however, that norepinephrine and serotonin dysfunctions merely reflect different aspects of the same fundamental illness. For example, when large doses of the norepinephrine precursor L-DOPA were administered to depressed patients, they showed some improvement in psychomotor retardation (activation) but no improvement in mood or cognition.[105] Similarly, L-tryptophan, the amino acid precursor of serotonin, has recently been shown to potentiate the effects of a tricyclic antidepressant on depressed mood and anxiety but not on the level of psychomotor activity or arousal.[106] These and other pharmacological data, taken as a whole, suggest that there may be some relationship betwen specific monoamine changes and distinct symptoms or clusters of symptoms. The finding that overall antidepressant response was dependent on adequate concentrations of both IMI (more serotonergic) and DMI (noradrenergic)[101] raises the possibility that in the absence of techniques to identify amine subgroups the more broad-spectrum antidepressant may represent the best choice for the treatment of affective illness. In this regard it is of interest that amitriptyline, considered by many to be the most effective of the tricyclics, should have the broadest spectrum of amine effects.

CONCLUSIONS

Any review of biological and pharmacological approaches to an understanding of affective illness inevitably raises questions as well as suggests answers. We have implicitly focused on two questions: first, whether we can learn more about the classification of affective illness through biological studies; second, whether we can improve pharmacotherapy by using biological predictors. Our answers are necessarily tentative because of the numerous methodological problems, particularly sources of variance, which we have discussed.

The combination of consistently abnormal monoamine metabolites levels, patterns of pharmacological response, and neuroendocrine correlates suggests that clear, biologically defined subgroups may eventually emerge. However the data on biological predictors need replication, and in light of the many sources of variance we should be very cautious in our interpretations. The use of these measures in practice is premature.

In order to evaluate the replicability and ultimate utility of these findings it will be necessary to conduct multivariant studies with large numbers of subjects. This will probably require different investigators' pooling data on a large number of variables collected under controlled conditions with standardized methods. The vast amount of data available from such a pool would allow the application of powerful computer-based multivariant statistical techniques able to deal with multiple sources of variance and multiple overlapping correlations. Such analyses could reveal associations between clusters of clinical findings, biochemical findings, and drug response findings that might alter our basic concepts about diagnostic categories or the mechanisms of action of various drugs. We may thereby support or refute the many provocative reports which already suggest practical implications for the management of affective illness. Future efforts will benefit from improved methods of clinical description and diagnosis, from more precise biological investigations, and from continued evaluations of pharmacological response.

REFERENCES

1. Winokur C, Clayton PJ, Reich T: *Manic-depressive Illness.* St. Louis, CV Mosby, 1969.
2. Gershon ES, Dunner DL, Goodwin FK: Toward a biology of affective illness: Genetic contributions. *Arch. Gen. Psychiatry 25:*1–15, 1971.
3. Grof P, Angst J, Haines T: The clinical course of depression: Practical issues. *Symposia Medica Hoechst 8:*141–148, 1973.
4. Klerman G: The long-term treatment of affective disorders. In: Lipton M, DiMascio A, Killam K (eds) *Psychopharmacology—A Generation of Progress.* New York, Raven Press, 1977.
5. Kendell RE: *The Classification of Depressive Illness.* London, Oxford University Press, 1968.
6. Goodwin FK: Diagnosis of affective disorders. In: Jarvik M (ed) *Psychopharmacology in the Practice of Medicine.* New York, Appleton-Century-Crofts, 1977.
7. Kiloh LH, Andrews G, Neilson M et al.: The relationship of the syndromes called endogenous and neurotic depression. *Br. J. Psychiatry 121:*183–196, 1972.
8. Paykel ES: Classification of depressed patients: A cluster analysis derived grouping. *Br. J. Psychiatry 118:*275–288, 1971.
9. Leff MJ, Roatch JF, Bunney WE Jr: Environmental factors preceding the onset of severe depressions. *Psychiatry 33:*293–311, 1970.
10. Paykel ES, Myers JK, Dieuelt MH et al.: Life events and depression. *Arch. Gen. Psychiatry 21:*753–760, 1969.
11. Kety SS: The central physiological and pharmacological effects of biogenic amines and their correlations with behavior. In: Quarton GC, Melnechuck T. Schmitt FO (eds) *The Neurosciences: A Study Program.* New York, Rockefeller University Press, 1967.
12. Cooper JR, Bloom FE, Roth RH: *The Biochemical Basis of Neuropharmacology.* Ed. II. New York, Oxford University Press, 1974.
13. Hockman CH, Bieger D (eds): *Chemical Transmission in the Mammalian Central Nervous System.* Baltimore, University Park Press, 1976.
14. Wurtman RJ: *Catecholamines.* Boston, Little, Brown, 1966.
15. Lemieux G, Davignon A, Genest J: Depressive states during Rauwolfia therapy for arterial hypertension: A report of 30 cases. *Can. Med. Assoc. J. 74:*522, 1956.
16. Ayd FJ: Thorazine and serpasil treatment of private neuropsychiatric patients. *Am. J. Psychiatry 113:*16, 1956.
17. Quetsch RM, Achor RWP, Litin EM et al.: Depressive reactions in hypertensive patients: A comparison of those treated with Rauwolfia and those receiving no specific antihypertensive treatment. *Circulation 19:*366, 1959.
18. Shore PA, Brodie BB: Influence of various drugs on serotonin and norepinephrine in the brain. In: Garattini S, Ghetti V (eds) *Psychotropic Drugs.* Amsterdam, Elsevier, 1957.
19. Carlsson A, Rosengren E, Bertler A et al.: Effect of reserpine on the metabolism of catecholamines. In: Garattini S, Ghetti V (eds) *Psychotropic Drugs.* Amsterdam, Elsevier, 1957.
20. Kline NS: Clinical experience with iproniazid (Marsilid). *J. Clin. Exp. Psychopath. 19:*72–78, 1958.
21. Davidson AN: Physiological role of monoamine oxidase. *Physiol. Rev. 38:*729–747, 1958.
22. Brodie BB, Spector S, Shore PA: Interaction of drugs with norepinephrine in the brain. *Pharmacol. Rev. 11:*548–564, 1959.

23. Prange AJ Jr: The use of drugs in depression: Its theoretical and practical basis. *Psychiatric Annals 3:*56–75, 1973.
24. Bunney WE Jr, Davis JM: Norepinephrine in depressive reactions. *Arch. Gen. Psychiatry 13:*483, 1965.
25. Schildkraut JJ: The catecholamine hypothesis of affective disorders: A review of supporting evidence. *Am. J. Psychiatry 122:*509, 1965.
26. Kuhn R: Über die Behandlung depressiver zustaende mit einem Iminodibenzylderivat (G22355). *Schweiz. Med. Wochenschr. 87:*1135–1140, 1957.
27. Carlsson, A, Corrodi H, Fuxe K et al.: Effects of some antidepressant drugs on the depletion of intraneuronal brain catecholamine stores caused by 4-*d*-dimethyl-meta-tyramine. *Europ. J. Pharmacol. 5:*367–373, 1969.
28. Glowinski J, Axelrod J: Inhibition of uptake of tritiated noradrenaline in the intact rat brain by imipramine and structurally related compounds. *Nature 204:*1318–1319, 1964.
29. Schou M: Special review: Lithium in psychiatric therapy and prophylaxis. *J. Psychiat. Res. 6:*67–95, 1968.
30. Colburn RW, Goodwin FK, Murphy DL et al.: Quantitative studies of norepinephrine uptake by synaptosomes. *Biochem. Pharmacol. 17:*957, 1968.
31. Katz RJ, Chase TN, Kopin IJ: Evoked release of norepinephrine and serotonin from brain slices: Inhibition by lithium. *Science 162:*466–467, 1968.
32. Maas JW: Biogenic amines and depression. *Arch. Gen. Psychiatry 32:*1357–1361, 1975.
33. Klein DF, Davis JM: *Diagnosis and Drug Treatment of Psychiatric Disorders*. Baltimore, Williams & Wilkins, 1969.
34. Post RM, Kotin J. Goodwin FK: Effects of cocaine in depressed patients. *Am. J. Psychiatry 131:*511–517, 1974.
35. Oswald I, Brezinova V, Dunleavy DLF: On the slowness of action of tricyclic antidepressant drugs. *Br. J. Psychiatry 120:*673–677, 1972.
36. Fann WE, Davis JM, Janowsky DS et al.: Effect of iprindole on amine uptake in man. *Arch. Gen. Psychiatry 26:*158–162, 1972.
37. Coppen A, Gupta RK, Montgomery S et al.: Mianserin hydrochloride: A novel antidepressant. *Br. J. Psychiatry 129:*342–345, 1976.
38. Ghose K, Coppen A, Turner P: Autonomic actions and interactions of mianserin hydrochloride (Org.GB.94) and amitriptyline in patients with depressive illness. *Psychopharmacology 49:*201–204, 1976.
39. Goodwin FK, Ebert M, Bunney WE Jr: Mental effects of reserpine in man. In: Shader RI (ed) *Psychiatric Complications of Medical Drugs*. New York, Raven Press, 1971.
40. Goodwin FK, Sack RL: Affective disorders: The catecholamine hypothesis revisited. In: Usdin E, Snyder S (eds) *Frontiers in Catecholamine Research*, pp. 1157–1164. New York, Pergamon Press, 1973.
41. Lovenberg W, Engelman K: Assay of serotonin, related metabolites and enzymes. *Meth. Biochem. Anal. 19:*1–34, 1971.
42. Vaughan GM, Pelham RW, Pang SF et al.: Nocturnal elevation of plasma melatonin and urinary 5-hydroxyindoleacetic acid in young men: Attempts at modification by brief changes in environmental lighting and sleep and by autonomic drugs. *J. Clin. Endocr. 42:*752–764, 1976.
43. Goodall McC, Alton H: Metabolism of 3-hydroxytryptamine (dopamine) in human subjects. *Biochem. Pharmacol. 17:*905–914, 1968.
44. Rinne UK, Sonninen U: Dopamine and Parkinson's disease. *Ann. Med. Intern. Fenn. 57:*105–113, 1968.
45. Weil–Malherbe H, van Buren JM: The excretion of dopamine and dopamine metabo-

lites in Parkinson's disease and the effect of diet thereon. *J. Lab. Clin. Med. 74:*305–318, 1969.

46. Calne DB, Karoum F, Ruthven CRJ et al.: The metabolism of orally administered L-DOPA in Parkinsonism. *Br. J. Pharmacol. 37:*57–68, 1969.
47. Tyce GM, Muenter MD, Owen CA Jr: Metabolism of L-dihydroxyphenylalanine by patients with Parkinson's disease. *Mayo. Clin. Proceedings 45:*645–656, 1970.
48. Goodall McC, Rosen L: Urinary excretion of noradrenaline and its metabolites at ten-minute intervals after intravenous injection of dl-Noradrenaline-2-C^{14}. *J. Clin. Invest. 42:*1578–1588, 1963.
49. Erwin GV: Oxidative-reductive pathways for metabolism of biogenic aldehydes. In: Usdin E (ed) *Frontiers of Catecholamine Research,* pp. 161–166. New York, Pergamon Press, 1973.
50. Maas JW, Landis DH: *In vitro* studies of the metabolism of norepinephrine in the central nervous system. *J. Pharmacol. Exp. Ther. 163:*147–162, 1968.
51. Maas JW, Dekirmenjian H, Garver D et al.: Excretion of catecholamine metabolites following intraventricular injection of 6-hydroxydopamine in the macaca speciosa. *Europ. J. Pharmacol. 23:*121–130, 1973.
52. Ebert M, Kopin IJ: Differential labeling of origins of urinary catecholamine metabolites by dopamine C^{14}. *Trans. Assoc. Amer. Physicians. 28:*256–264, 1975.
53. Maas JW, Fawcett JA, Dekirmenjian H: 3-Methoxy-4-hydroxyphenylglycol (MHPG) execretion in depressive patients: A pilot study. *Arch. Gen. Psychiatry 19:*129–134, 1968.
54. Greenspan K, Schildkraut JJ, Gordon EK et al.: Catecholamine metabolism in affective disorders. III. MHPG and other catecholamine metabolites in patients treated with lithium carbonate. *J. Psychiat. Res. 7:*171–183, 1970.
55. Bond PA, Jenner FA, Sampson GA: Daily variations of the urine content of 3-methoxy-4-hydroxyphenylglycol in two manic-depressive patients. *Psychol. Med. 2:*81–85, 1972.
56. Jones DF, Maas JW, Dekirmenjian H et al.: Urinary catecholamine metabolites during behavioral changes in a patient with manic-depressive cycles. *Science 179:*300–302, 1973.
57. Stoddard FJ, Post RM, Gillin JC et al.: Phasic changes in manic-depressive illness. Presented at the annual meeting, American Psychiatric Association, Detroit, Michigan, May 1974.
58. Muscettola G, Wehr T, Goodwin FK: Central norepinephrine responses in depression versus normals. Presented at the annual meeting, American Psychiatric Association, *New Research Abstracts,* p. 8, Miami, Florida, May 1976.
59. Gordon EK, Perlow M, Oliver J et al.: Origins of catecholamine metabolites in monkey cerebrospinal fluid. *J. Neurochem. 25:*347–349, 1975.
60. Karoum F, Gillin JC, Wyatt RJ: Mass fragmentographic determination of some acidic and alcoholic metabolites of biogenic amines in the rat brain. *J. Neurochem. 25:*653–658, 1975.
61. Goodwin FK, Post RM: Studies of amine metabolites in affective illness and in schizophrenia: A comparative analysis. In: Freedman DX (ed) *The Biology of the Major Psychoses.* Vol. 54, pp. 299–332. New York, Raven Press, 1975.
62. Moir ATB, Ashcroft GW, Crawford TBB et al.: Central metabolites in cerebrospinal fluid as a biochemical approach to the brain. *Brain 93:*357–368, 1970.
63. Gordon EK, Oliver J, Goodwin FK et al.: Effect of probenecid on free 3-methoxy-4-hydroxyphenylethylene glycol (MHPG) and its sulfate in human cerebrospinal fluid. *Neuropharmacol. 12:*391–396, 1973.

64. Korf J, van Praag HM: Amine metabolites in the human brain: Further evaluation of the probenecid test. *Brain Res. 35:*221–230, 1971.
65. Sjostrom R: Steady-state levels of probenecid and their relation to acid monoamine metabolites in human cerebrospinal fluid. *Psychopharmacologia (Berl.) 25:*96–100, 1972.
66. Bowers MB Jr: Fluorometric measurement of 5-hydroxyindoleacetic acid (5HIAA) and tryptophan in human CSF: Effects of high doses of probenecid. *Biol. Psychiat. 9:*93–97, 1974.
67. Perel JM, Levitt M, Dunner DL: Plasma and cerebrospinal fluid probenecid concentrations as related to accumulation of acidic biogenic amine metabolites in man. *Psychopharmacology 35:*83–90, 1974.
68. Ebert MH, Cowdry RW, Goodwin FK et al.: Unpublished manuscript, 1977.
69. Subrahmanyan S: Role of biogenic amines in certain pathological conditions. *Brain Res. 87:*355–362, 1975.
70. Asberg M, Thoren P, Traskman L et al.: "Serotonin depression"—A biochemical subgroup within the affective disorders? *Science 191:*478–480, 1976.
71. Goodwin FK, Wehr T, Post RM: Clinical approaches to the evaluation of brain amine function in mental illness: Some conceptual issues. In: Lovenberg, Youdim (eds) *Essays in Neurochemistry and Neuropharmacology,* Vol. 2, pp. 71–104. London, John Wiley & Sons, 1977.
72. Lapin IP, Oxenkrug GF: Intensification of the central serotonergic processes as a possible determinant of the thymoleptic effect. *Lancet i:*132–136, 1969.
73. Coppen AJ, Prange AJ Jr, Whybrow PC et al.: Abnormalities of indoleamines in affective disorders. *Arch. Gen. Psychiatry 26:*474–478, 1972.
74. Goodwin FK, Beckmann H: Urinary MHPG in unipolar and bipolar affective disorders. *Sci. Proc. Am. Psychiat. Assoc. 128:*96–97, 1975.
75. Maas JW, Dekiremenjian H, Jones F: The identification of depressed patients who have a disorder of NE metabolism and/or disposition. In: Usdin E, Snyder S (eds) *Frontiers in Catecholamine Research,* pp. 1091–1096. New York, Pergamon Press, 1973.
76. Klerman GL, Cole JC: Clinical pharmacology of imipramine and related antidepressant compounds. *Pharmacol. Rev. 17:*101–141, 1965.
77. Sjoqvist FB: A pharmacokinetic approach to the treatment of depression. *Int. Pharmacopsychiatry 6:*147–169, 1971.
78. Biggs JT, Chang SS, Sherman WR et al.: Measurement of tricyclic antidepressant levels in an outpatient clinic. *J. Nerv. Ment. Dis. 162:*46–51, 1976.
79. Asberg M, Cronholm B, Sjoqvist FB et al.: Relationship between plasma level and therapeutic effect of nortriptyline. *Br. Med. J. III:*331–334, 1971.
80. Kragh-Sorensen P, Hansen CE, Baastrup PC et al.: Self-inhibiting action of nortriptylin's antidepressive effect at high plasma levels. *Psychopharmacologia 45:*305–312, 1976.
81. Ziegler VE, Clayton PJ, Taylor JR et al.: Nortriptyline plasma levels and therapeutic response. *Clin. Pharmacol. Ther. 20:*458–463, 1976.
82. Leonhard K: *Aufteilung der Endogenen Psychosen.* ed. II. Berlin, 1959.
83. Goodwin FK, Muscettola G, Gold PW et al.: Biochemical and pharmacological differentiation of affective disorder. In: Akiskal H, Webb W (eds) *Psychiatric Diagnoses: Exploration of Biological Criteria.* New York, Plenum Press, in press.
84. Schildkraut J, Keeler BA, Grob EL et al.: MHPG excretion and clinical classification in depression. *Lancet i:*1251–1252, 1973.
85. Spitzer RL, Endicott J, Robbins E: Research Diagnostic Criteria. *Psychopharmacol. Bull. 11:*22–25, 1975.
86. Goodwin FK, Cowdry R, Jimmerson D et al.: Serotonin and norepinephrine "sub-

groups" in depression: Metabolite findings and clinical-pharmacological correlations. *Sci. Proc. Amer. Psychiat. Assn. 130:*108, 1977.

87. Goodwin FK, Cowdry R, Webster M: Predictors of pharmacological efficacy in the affective disorders. In: Lipton M. DiMascio A, Killam K (eds) *Psychopharmacology—A Generation of Progress.* New York, Raven Press, 1977.
88. Asberg M, Trajksman L, Thoren P: 5-HIAA in the cerebrospinal fluid. *Arch. Gen. Psychiatry 33:*1193–1197, 1976.
89. Frohman LA, Strachura ME: Neuropharmacologic control of neuroendocrine function by man. *Metabolism 24:*211–233, 1975.
90. Sachar EJ (ed): *Hormones, Behavior and Psychopathology.* New York, Raven Press, 1976.
91. Carroll BJ, Curtis GG, Mendels J: Neuroendocrine regulation in depression. *Arch. Gen. Psychiatry 33:*1039–1044, 1976.
92. Gold PW, Goodwin FK: Urinary free cortisol in depression and mania. Presented at the Annual Meeting of the American Psychiatric Association, Toronto, Ontario, Canada, May 1977.
93. Gold P, Goodwin FK, Wehr T, et al.: Thyrotropin response to thyrotropin releasing hormone in affective illness: Correlation with CSF amine metabolites *Am. J. Psychiatry,* 1977 (in press).
94. Yoshimura M, Ochi Y, Miyazaki T et al.: Effect of L-5-HTP on release of growth hormone, TSH and insulin. *Endocrinol. Jap. 20:*135, 1973.
95. Bertilsson L, Asberg M, Thoren P: Differential effect of chlorimipramine and nortriptyline on cerebrospinal fluid metabolites of serotonin and noradrenaline in depression. *Europ. J. Clin. Pharmacol. 7:*365–368, 1974.
96. Asberg M, Ringberger VA, Sjoqvist F et al.: Monoamine metabolites in cerebrospinal fluid and serotonin uptake inhibition during treatment with chlorimipramine. *Clin. Pharm. Ther. 21:*201–207, 1977.
97. Muscettola G, Goodwin FK, Potter WZ, et al.: Imipramine and desipramine in plasma and spinal fluid: Relationship to clinical response and serotonin metabolism. *Arch. Gen. Psychiatry,* 1977 (in press).
98. Sathananthan GL, Gershon S, Almeida M et al.: Correlation between plasma and cerebrospinal levels of imipramine. *Arch. Gen. Psychiatry 33:*1109–1110, 1976.
99. Carlsson A, Corrodi H, Fuxe K et al.: Effect of some antidepressant drugs on the depletion of intraneuronal brain 5-hydroxytryptamine stores caused by 4-methyl-alpha-ethyl-meta-tyramine. *Europ. J. Pharmacol. 5:*357–366, 1969.
100. Hamberger B, Tuck JR: Effect of tricyclic antidepressants on the uptake of noradrenaline and 5-hydroxytryptamine by rat brain slices incubated in buffer or human plasma. *Europ. J. Clin. Pharmacol. 5:*229–235, 1973.
101. Gram LF, Reisby N, Ibsen I et al.: Plasma levels and antidepressive effect of imipramine. *Clin. Pharmacol. Ther. 19*(3):318–324, 1976.
102. Ziegler VE, Co BU, Taylor JR et al.: Amitriptyline plasma levels and therapeutic response. *Clin. Pharm. Ther. 19:*795–801, 1976.
103. Asberg M, Bertilsson L, Tuck JR et al.: Indoleamine metabolites in the cerebrospinal fluid of depressed patients before and during treatment with nortriptyline. *Clin. Pharm. Ther. 14:*277–286, 1973.
104. Siwers B, Ringberger VA, Tuck JR et al.: Initial clinical trial based on biochemical methodology of Zimelidine (a serotonin uptake inhibitor) in depressed patients. *Clin. Pharm. Ther. 21:*194–200, 1977.
105. Goodwin FK, Brodie HKH, Murphy DL et al.: L-DOPA, catecholamines and behavior: A clinical and biochemical study in depressed patients. *Biol. Psychiatry 2:*341–366, 1970.

106. Carlsson A: The influence of antidepressants on central monoaminergic systems. In: van Praag (ed) *Neurotransmission and Disturbed Behavior*. Amsterdam, Bohn BV, 1977.

3

Norepinephrine Metabolism in Depressive Disorders: Implications for a Biochemical Classification of Depressions

JOSEPH J. SCHILDKRAUT, PAUL J. ORSULAK, JON E. GUDEMAN, ALAN F. SCHATZBERG, WILLIAM A. ROHDE, RICHARD A. LABRIE, JANE F. CAHILL, JONATHAN O. COLE, and SHERVERT H. FRAZIER

The introduction of drugs (e.g., monoamine oxidase inhibitor antidepressants, tricyclic antidepressants and lithium salts) which proved to be effective in the treatment of depressive and manic disorders has had a major impact not only on clinical psychiatric practice but also on biological research in psychiatry. The neuropharmacology of these drugs has been studied extensively by a large number of investigators and the findings of these studies suggest that the effects of these drugs on the metabolism of the biogenic amines (i.e., the catecholamines, norepinephrine, and dopamine, as well as the indoleamine, serotonin) may be of importance clinically.[1] These neuropharmacological findings served to stimulate considerable interest in biological research in the affective disorders, and many clues to the underlying pathophysiology of depressive and manic disorders have emerged from this research in recent years.[2]

The clinical and biological heterogeneity of the depressive disorders has long been recognized among psychiatrists, and the possibility that different subgroups of patients with depressive disorders might be characterized by differences in the metabolism of one or another

JOSEPH J. SCHILDKRAUT ET AL. • Department of Psychiatry, Harvard Medical School; Neuropsychopharmacology Laboratory, Massachusetts Mental Health Center, Boston, Massachusetts; and McLean Hospital, Belmont, Massachusetts.

monoamine was suggested more than ten years ago in a review of the catecholamine hypothesis of affective disorders.[3] Recent studies by our group and others have explored this possibility, and preliminary findings now indicate that biochemical measures related to biogenic amine metabolism may provide a basis for classifying depressive disorders and possibly also for predicting differential antidepressant responses to various forms of treatment. This paper will summarize selected aspects of our recent research on catecholamine metabolism in the affective disorders, emphasizing those findings which suggest that the differences in norepinephrine metabolism in patients with depressive disorders may be useful biochemical criteria for distinguishing different types of depressions.

REVIEW OF INITIAL STUDIES OF NORMETANEPHRINE EXCRETION AND AFFECTIVE STATE

A number of years ago, the now classic studies of norepinephrine metabolism performed by Axelrod, Kopin, and their associates suggested that normetanephrine, the *O*-methylated metabolite of norepinephrine, might derive from norepinephrine that was released from presynaptic neurons into the synaptic cleft where it could interact with postsynaptic receptor sites.[4–6] It was, therefore, of interest to us to examine the excretion of normetanephrine in our early longitudinal studies of the changes in norepinephrine metabolism that occur in association with changes in affective state in depressive and manic disorders.[7] In these studies we found that the excretion of normetanephrine, the metabolite of norepinephrine that may best reflect the level of norepinephrine present extraneuronally and available to receptors, was relatively lower during periods of depression and relatively higher during periods of hypomania as compared to levels during periods of normal affective state in some, but not all, patients with affective disorders. In these studies, we also observed a gradual increase in normetanephrine excretion during the period of definitive clinical improvement in depressed patients treated with the tricyclic antidepressant drug imipramine. This finding has been confirmed by other investigators.[8,9] However, the urinary excretion of normetanephrine may primarily reflect the activity of the peripheral sympathetic nervous system, since it is probable that only a small fraction of urinary normetanephrine or norepinephrine derives from the brain because of the relatively effective brain-blood barrier to these monoamines.[10,11]

MHPG: A METABOLITE OF BRAIN NOREPINEPHRINE

It was, therefore, of interest to us, some years ago, to examine the metabolism of normetanephrine within the central nervous system. In these studies, we found that normetanephrine (as well as norepinephrine) was principally metabolized to the sulfate conjugate of 3-methoxy-4-hydroxyphenylglycol (MHPG) in the rat brain[12]; and we subsequently identified MHPG and its sulfate conjugate in human cerebrospinal fluid.[13] Concurrently, other investigators showed that in dogs most norepinephrine originating in the brain was excreted in the urine as MHPG,[14] and in a pilot study[15] they reported that MHPG excretion was reduced in depressed patients. Other findings also suggest that in several different species, including man, MHPG or its sulfate conjugate is the major metabolite of norepinephrine in the brain,[16–18] but all findings do not concur.[19] MHPG, which is excreted in the urine, may also come, in part, from the peripheral sympathetic nervous system,[20] and the fraction of urinary MHPG which in fact derives from norepinephrine originating in the brain remains problematic.[21,22] However, recent data suggest that, in man, the contribution from the brain may be substantial—i.e., greater than 50%.[23]

MHPG EXCRETION AND AFFECTIVE STATE IN NATURALLY OCCURRING OR AMPHETAMINE-INDUCED MANIC-DEPRESSIVE EPISODES

In one aspect of our research we have examined the changes in MHPG excretion which were associated with changes in affective state. The findings from our longitudinal studies of individual patients with naturally occurring or amphetamine-induced manic-depressive (i.e., bipolar) episodes indicate that levels of urinary MHPG are relatively lower during depressions and higher during manic or hypomanic episodes than after clinical remissions,[24–27] and these findings have been confirmed by other investigators[28,29] but not by all.[30,31]

The relationship between MHPG excretion and clinical state that we have observed in manic-depressive (i.e., bipolar) patients is illustrated in Figure 1, which summarizes the changes in MHPG excretion in a manic-depressive patient studied longitudinally through five successive drug-free periods which were defined by differences in clinical state. During the initial period summarized here, the patient was mildly depressed. Following this, there was a decrease in MHPG excretion and the patient became severely depressed. During treatment with electroconvulsive shock (ECT), there was a gradual increase in MHPG excretion and the depression gradually subsided. Following ECT, there was a further increase in MHPG excretion and the patient became transiently hypomanic. Subsequently, there was a decrease in MHPG excretion as the hypomania subsided and the patient again became mildly depressed. These data show the close association between MHPG excretion and changes in affective state which we observed in patients with bipolar manic-depressive disorders.

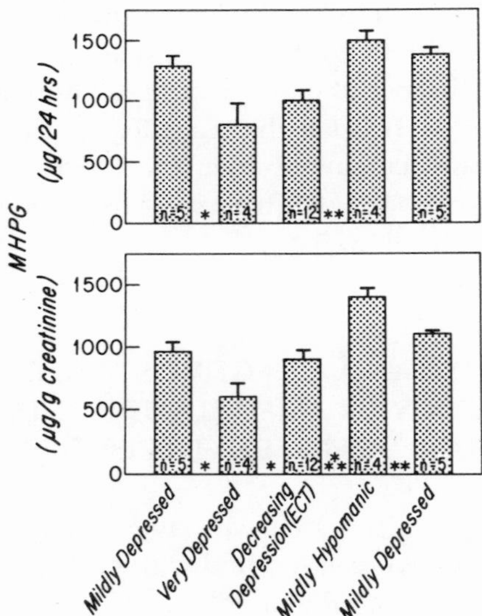

Figure 1. MHPG excretion and affective state in a manic-depressive patient. MHPG excretion was determined in a bipolar manic-depressive patient studied through five successive drug-free periods that were defined by differences in clinical state. MHPG is expressed both in μg/24 hours and μg/g creatinine. N = number of urine samples analyzed in each period. $^{*}p < 0.05$; $^{**}p < 0.001$; $^{***}p < 0.001$ for differences in MHPG between adjacent periods. (Data from Schildkraut et al.[25])

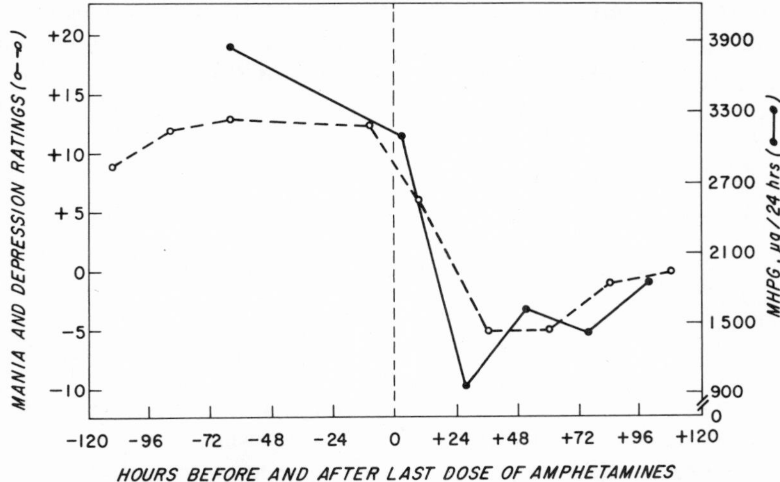

Figure 2. Clinical state and MHPG excretion before and after withdrawal of amphetamines. The last dose of amphetamines was taken at 0 hours. Each value for MHPG was plotted at the midpoint of the 24-hour urine collection period. Each clinical rating was plotted at the midpoint of the 24-hour period covered by that rating. Mania ratings (+). Depression ratings (−). (Reproduced from Schildkraut et al.[26])

Figure 2 shows the changes in MHPG excretion and clinical state in one of four amphetamine abusers studied during the course of amphetamine withdrawal. While still taking high doses of amphetamines, the patient showed elevated MHPG excretion and was clinically hypomanic (as evidenced by the positive scores on the mania–depression rating scale). Upon abrupt withdrawal of amphetamines, there was a prompt fall in MHPG excretion and the patient became depressed (as evidenced by the negative scores on the mania–depression rating scale). Starting about 48 hours after amphetamine withdrawal, there was a gradual increase in MHPG excretion accompanied by a gradual remission of the depression. Thus, in patients with amphetamine-induced manic-depressive oscillations, we also saw a close association between MHPG excretion and affective state.[26,27]

Thus, in longitudinal studies of MHPG excretion in patients with bipolar manic-depressive disorders, we have observed that MHPG excretion was relatively lower during depressions and relatively higher during hypomanias than during periods of clinical remission. However, all depressions are not clinically or biologically homogeneous,[3] and all depressed patients do not excrete comparably low levels of

MHPG.[9] Our recent research has, therefore, explored the possibility that the urinary excretion of MHPG and other catecholamine metabolites might provide a biochemical basis for differentiating among the depressive disorders.

INITIAL STUDY OF DIFFERENCES IN MHPG EXCRETION IN CLINICALLY DEFINED SUBTYPES OF DEPRESSIVE DISORDERS

In our initial preliminary study,[32,33] we examined MHPG excretion in a small group of patients with certain clinically defined subtypes of depressive disorders.[34] All patients were studied during a period of clinical depression at a time when they were receiving no psychoactive drugs. Since we had found MHPG excretion to vary with clinical state in bipolar manic-depressive disorders, we were particularly interested in comparing MHPG excretion in bipolar manic-depressive depressions and in other clinically defined types of depressive disorders that might represent biologically different entities. Because most bipolar manic-depressive depressions present as endogenous depressive syndromes and it is most unusual for bipolar patients to show chronic characterological depressive syndromes (i.e., dysphoric depressive syndromes), unipolar chronic characterological depressions were selected as the principal comparison group in this initial study. This was done in order to minimize the likelihood of having patients with clinically latent bipolar disorders (i.e., bipolar patients who had not yet manifested their first hypomanic or manic episode) in the comparison group.

As shown in Figure 3, in this initial study of 12 patients we found that MHPG excretion was significantly lower in 5 patients with bipolar manic-depressive depressions than in 5 patients with unipolar chronic characterological depressions. We also observed low MHPG excretion in one patient with a schizoaffective depression and, in addition, intermediate levels of MHPG in one patient with a unipolar recurrent endogenous depression.[32,33]

Because it had been suggested that differences in physical activity or stress could conceivably account for the differences in MHPG excretion observed in patients with affective disorders,[35–37] we examined our data in several different ways for possible relationships between MHPG excretion and clinical assessments of motor activity and anxiety as re-

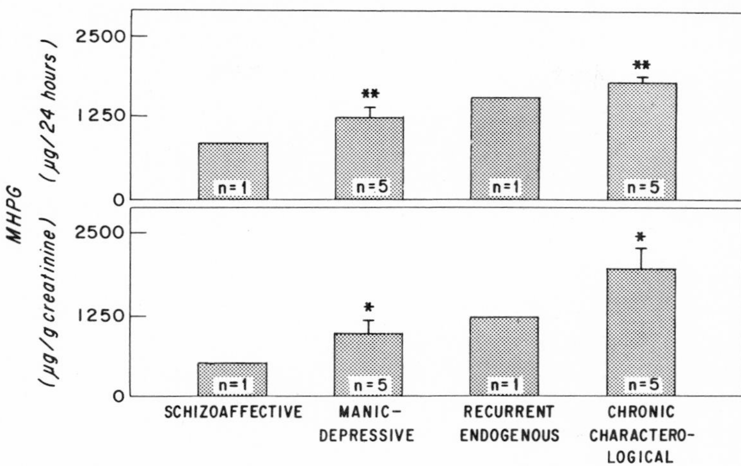

Figure 3. MHPG excretion in depressive disorders. MHPG was determined in 3 to 10 separate 24-hour urine samples from each patient. These individual values were averaged to obtain an overall value for each subject; this value was then used in computing the means and standard errors of the means for the two groups (manic-depressive and chronic characterological depressions). $^{*}p < 0.05$; $^{**}p < 0.02$ for difference between manic-depressive and chronic characterological depressions. (Reproduced from Schildkraut et al.[33])

flected by scores on a modified Hamilton Depression Rating Scale.[38] As shown in Table I, there were no significant differences in scores for retardation, agitation, and psychic or somatic anxiety between the manic-depressive and chronic characterological depressions. Moreover, when the entire group of 12 depressed patients were subdivided into the 4 with lowest, the 4 with intermediate, and the 4 with highest scores on each of these items, no corresponding differences in MHPG excretion emerged (Tables II and III). There were also no meaningful correlations between MHPG excretion and scores for retardation, agitation, and

TABLE I. HAMILTON DEPRESSION RATING SCALE ITEMS IN MANIC-DEPRESSIVE AND CHRONIC CHARACTEROLOGICAL DEPRESSIONS[a]

Hamilton item	Manic-depressive	Chronic characterological	p
Retardation	0.75 ± 0.28	0.59 ± 0.20	n.s.
Agitation	1.01 ± 0.17	1.20 ± 0.06	n.s.
Anxiety (psychic)	2.50 ± 0.15	2.44 ± 0.18	n.s.
Anxiety (somatic)	0.80 ± 0.34	1.08 ± 0.42	n.s.

[a]Reproduced from Schildkraut.[39]

TABLE II. MHPG EXCRETION IN DEPRESSIVE DISORDERS WITH LOW AND HIGH RETARDATION OR AGITATION[a]

	H.D.R.S.[b] score	MHPG (μg/day)
Retardation		
Low (N = 4)	0.21 ± .09	1510 ± 280
Middle (N = 4)	0.49 ± .03	1290 ± 180
High (N = 4)	1.24 ± .10	1620 ± 160
Agitation		
Low (N = 4)	0.77 ± .10	1510 ± 150
Middle (N = 4)	1.16 ± .01	1510 ± 70
High (N = 4)	1.44 ± .06	1390 ± 360

[a]Reproduced from Schildkraut.[39]
[b]H.D.R.S. = Hamilton Depression Rating Scale.

psychic or somatic anxiety (Table IV). (See reference 39.) Other investigators have recently made similar observations concerning the absence of an association between MHPG excretion and marked retardation or agitation in depressed patients.[40] These findings thus provide no support for the suggestion that differences in MHPG excretion in patients with affective disorders reflect only differences in activity or stress.

In interpreting these data, one cannot exclude the possibility that these Hamilton Depression Rating Scale items were not specific or sensitive enough to detect differences in retardation, agitation, or anxiety

TABLE III. MHPG EXCRETION IN DEPRESSIVE DISORDERS WITH LOW AND HIGH ANXIETY[a]

	H.D.R.S.[b] score	MHPG (μg/day)
Anxiety (psychic)		
Low (N = 4)	2.11 ± .01	1510 ± 140
Middle (N = 4)	2.40 ± .12	1400 ± 210
High (N = 4)	2.83 ± .07	1500 ± 290
Anxiety (somatic)		
Low (N = 4)	0.22 ± .08	1440 ± 120
Middle (N = 4)	0.83 ± .15	1460 ± 200
High (N = 4)	1.83 ± .17	1510 ± 320

[a]Reproduced from Schildkraut.[39]
[b]H.D.R.S. = Hamilton Depression Rating Scale.

TABLE IV. CORRELATIONS BETWEEN HAMILTON DEPRESSION RATING SCALE ITEMS AND MHPG EXCRETION[a]

Hamilton item	Correlation coefficient	p
Retardation	0.24	n.s.
Agitation	−0.19	n.s.
Anxiety (psychic)	−0.19	n.s.
Anxiety (somatic)	0.11	n.s.

[a]Reproduced from Schildkraut.[39]

which may have been related to MHPG excretion. However, this possibility is weakened by the fact that we did observe meaningful relationships between several of these Hamilton Depression Rating Scale items and certain other biochemical variables. For example, patients with high scores on retardation excreted significantly less epinephrine and tended to excrete less metanephrine than patients with lower retardation scores, whereas patients with higher scores on somatic anxiety excreted significantly more metanephrine than did patients with low scores on this item (Tables V and VI).

We also examined our data for possible differences between the bipolar manic-depressive and unipolar chronic characterological depressions, as evidenced by scores on other items of the Hamilton Depression Rating Scale[38] or the Mania–Depression Rating Scale.[41] While there were no significant differences in total depression rating scores between these groups, patients with unipolar chronic characterological depressions tended to have higher scores on hypochondriasis, dramatic atten-

TABLE V. EPINEPHRINE EXCRETION IN DEPRESSIVE DISORDERS WITH LOW AND HIGH RETARDATION

Retardation	H.D.R.S.[a] score	Epinephrine (μg/day)
Low (N = 4)	0.21 ± .09	13 ± 3[b]
Middle (N = 4)	0.49 ± .03	12 ± 3
High (N = 4)	1.24 ± .10	6 ± 1[b]

[a]H.D.R.S. = Hamilton Depression Rating Scale.
[b]$p < 0.05$ (one-tailed) for difference between groups with low and high retardation scores.

tion seeking, and items related to sleep disturbances. These findings, of course, may simply reflect the clinical criteria used to define the chronic characterological depressive syndrome, which include hypochondriasis and dramatic attention seeking[34]; but they, nonetheless, support the notion that a different clinical syndrome occurs in bipolar manic-depressive depressions (classified simply on the basis of a prior history of mania or hypomania).

The differences in Hamilton Depression Rating Scale scores for early, middle, and late insomnia, as well as average insomnia, are shown in Table VII. While patients with unipolar chronic characterological depressions tended to report more disturbances of sleep throughout the night than did patients with bipolar manic-depressive depressions, these differences were most pronounced in the later part of the night. These preliminary findings of relatively more reported insomnia in patients with unipolar chronic characterological depressions than in patients with bipolar manic-depressive depressions seem consistent with other studies of sleep patterns in patients with bipolar manic-depressive depressions.[42–44]

Data from all-night electroencephalographic sleep recordings (performed by Dr. Ernest Hartmann) tended to support these differences in Hamilton Depression Rating Scale scores of sleep disturbances based on patients' reports. Although none of the electroencephalographically recorded variables showed statistically significant differences in this small series, patients with unipolar chronic characterological depressions did tend to have longer sleep latencies, shorter total sleep time, and more waking time than did patients with bipolar manic-depressive depressions.

TABLE VI. METANEPHRINE EXCRETION IN DEPRESSIVE DISORDERS WITH LOW AND HIGH SOMATIC ANXIETY

Somatic anxiety	H.D.R.S.[a] score	Metanephrine (μg/day)
Low (N = 4)	0.22 ± .08	117 ± 5[b]
Middle (N = 4)	0.83 ± .15	203 ± 22
High (N = 4)	1.83 ± .17	218 ± 33[b]

[a]H.D.R.S. = Hamilton Depression Rating Scale.
[b]$p < 0.02$ (one-tailed) for difference between groups with low and high somatic anxiety scores.

TABLE VII. H.D.R.S.[a] INSOMNIA RATINGS IN MANIC-DEPRESSIVE AND CHRONIC CHARACTEROLOGICAL DEPRESSIONS

Hamilton item	Manic-depressive	Chronic characterological	p
Early insomnia	1.22 ± 0.34	1.54 ± 0.17	n.s.
Middle insomnia	0.90 ± 0.31	1.62 ± 0.11	.09
Late insomnia	0.92 ± 0.32	1.90 ± 0.09	.03
Average insomnia[b]	1.01 ± 0.27	1.69 ± 0.10	.07

[a]H.D.R.S. = Hamilton Depression Rating Scale.
[b]Average insomnia = the average of the scores for early, middle, and late insomnia.

REPLICATION STUDY OF MHPG AS A BIOCHEMICAL CRITERION FOR CLASSIFYING DEPRESSIVE DISORDERS

We have subsequently replicated and extended our findings of differences in MHPG excretion in different subtypes of depressive disorders in another series of 25 depressed patients with clearcut schizoaffective, bipolar manic-depressive, unipolar endogenous, unipolar chronic characterological, or unipolar nonspecific depressive syndromes.* (Excluded were patients with histories of chronic asocial or eccentric behaviors, patients with histories of amphetamine or barbiturate abuse, and patients with depressions that could not be uniquely classified according to our system for classifying depressive disorders.) Since MHPG excretion was comparably reduced in patients with schizoaffective and bipolar manic-depressive depressions, these two groups were combined in the analysis of data. Similarly, since there were no differences in MHPG excretion in patients with unipolar chronic characterological or unipolar nonspecific depressions, these two groups were combined for the purposes of data analysis.

Table VIII presents the data on MHPG excretion in the initial sample of 12 patients (summarized in Figure 3), the replication sample of 25 patients, and the total sample of 37 patients. As shown in Table VIII, the replication sample also showed significantly lower MHPG excretion in the schizoaffective and bipolar manic-depressive depressions than in the unipolar chronic characterological and unipolar nonspecific depressions. Considering the total sample of 37 depressed patients, we found that 13

*The term *unipolar nonspecific depressive syndrome* is used to refer to unipolar depressive disorders that fit no specific syndrome (e.g., endogenous or chronic characterological) in our nosological system.[34]

TABLE VIII. MHPG[a] EXCRETION IN DEPRESSIVE DISORDERS

Sample	Bipolar manic-depressive and schizoaffective	Unipolar endogenous	Unipolar chronic characterological and nonspecific
Initial	1176 ± 145 (N = 6)	1551 (N = 1)	1803 ± 89[c] (N = 5)
Replication	1235 ± 98 (N = 9)	1728 ± 196[b] (N = 8)	1821 ± 152[c] (N = 8)
Total	1211 ± 80 (N = 15)	1709 ± 174[d] (N = 9)	1814 ± 96[d] (N = 13)

[a]MHPG was determined in 2 to 10 separate 24-hour urine samples obtained from each patient. The average value for each patient was used to compute the group means and standard errors of the means presented in this table. MHPG is expressed in μg per 24 hours. N = number of patients.
[b]$p < 0.05$, [c]$p < 0.01$, [d]$p < 0.001$ for comparisons between bipolar manic-depressive and schizoaffective group versus unipolar chronic characterological and nonspecific groups, or unipolar endogenous group.

of the 15 patients with schizoaffective or bipolar manic-depressive depressions had MHPG levels less than 1500 μg/day, whereas in 12 of the 13 patients with unipolar chronic characterological or unipolar nonspecific depressions the levels of MHPG were 1500 μg/day or higher.

While the mean MHPG excretion in the group of unipolar endogenous depressions was higher than in the group of schizoaffective and bipolar manic-depressive depressions, 3 of the 9 patients with unipolar endogenous depressions had MHPG levels below 1500 μg/day. This suggests that the group that we identify clinically as unipolar endogenous depressions may be biochemically heterogeneous, with some patients in this group bearing a biochemical similarity to the schizoaffective and bipolar manic-depressive depressions. (As noted above, one might expect that some of the patients, classified as unipolar because there was no prior history of hypomania or mania, might subsequently become hypomanic or manic, particularly when the disorder presents as an endogenous depressive syndrome.)

The highly significant differences ($p < 0.001$) in MHPG excretion between the schizoaffective and bipolar manic-depressive depressions versus the unipolar chronic characterological and nonspecific depressions could not be explained by sex differences, since the various diagnostic groups were reasonably balanced with respect to sex distribution (Table IX). Moreover, as shown in Table IX, there were no significant differences in age, severity of depression (assessed on the modified Hamilton Depression Rating Scale),[38] urine volume, or creatinine excretion.

TABLE IX. SEX, AGE, HAMILTON DEPRESSION RATINGS, URINE VOLUME, AND CREATININE IN DEPRESSIVE DISORDERS

	Bipolar manic-depressive and schizoaffective	Unipolar endogenous	Unipolar chronic characterological and nonspecific
Sex (M/F)	7/8	5/4	7/6
Age (years)	38 ± 3	46 ± 5	42 ± 4
Hamilton depression ratings	32 ± 2	28 ± 3	30 ± 2
Urine volume (ml/24 hours)	1080 ± 108	1129 ± 211	983 ± 74
Creatinine (mg/24 hours)	1248 ± 113	1215 ± 146	1100 ± 66

We also measured the urinary excretion of norepinephrine, normetanephrine, epinephrine, metanephrine, and 3-methoxy-4-hydroxymandelic acid (VMA) in these patients. As indicated in Table X, the urinary excretion of norepinephrine tended to be lower in schizoaffective and bipolar manic-depressive depressions than in the unipolar endogenous depressions or unipolar chronic characterological and nonspecific depressions; but these differences were only of borderline statistical significance. There were no other statistically significant differences in normetanephrine, epinephrine, metanephrine, or VMA excretion among these diagnostic groups of depressive disorders (Table X). Thus, of the

TABLE X. NOREPINEPHRINE, NORMETANEPHRINE, EPINEPHRINE, METANEPHRINE, AND VMA IN DEPRESSIVE DISORDERS

	Bipolar manic-depressive and schizoaffective	Unipolar endogenous	Unipolar chronic characterological and nonspecific
Norepinephrine (μg/24 hours)	27 ± 3	41 ± 6	39 ± 6
Normetanephrine (μg/24 hours)	237 ± 24	315 ± 51	247 ± 28
Epinephrine (μg/24 hours)	9 ± 1	10 ± 2	10 ± 2
Metanephrine (μg/24 hours)	174 ± 16	151 ± 15	168 ± 16
VMA (μg/24 hours)	4022 ± 187	3616 ± 280	3583 ± 222

urinary catecholamines and metabolites that we measured, only MHPG showed highly significant differences among the subgroups of depressive disorders.

Our findings on the relationship between MHPG excretion and the clinical classification of depressive disorders have recently been supported by the work of two other groups of investigators, although somewhat different systems of classification were used in each of these studies. Goodwin and his associates[45] have confirmed our findings of relatively lower MHPG excretion in bipolar depressions than in unipolar depressions; and similar findings of low MHPG in patients with bipolar depressions have been reported by Maas and Jones and their associates.[40,46] The relative lowering of MHPG excretion in schizoaffective and bipolar manic-depressive depressions may be related to the recent observations that platelet monoamine oxidase activity was decreased in patients with some types of schizophrenias,[47,48] as well as in patients with bipolar manic-depressive disorders,[49] but relatively increased in other types of depressive disorders.[50]

In summary, our findings suggest that there may be a biologically related group of depressive disorders with relatively low MHPG excretion (of which bipolar manic-depressive depressions represent a clinically identifiable subgroup) and a biologically related group of depressive disorders with relatively high MHPG excretion (of which unipolar chronic characterological depressions represent a clinically identifiable subgroup). Thus, our findings support the possibility that the distinction between depressions with relatively low and high MHPG excretion may provide a biochemical criterion for classifying the depressive disorders.

PRELIMINARY STUDY OF PRETREATMENT MHPG EXCRETION AS A PREDICTOR OF THE ANTIDEPRESSANT RESPONSE TO AMITRIPTYLINE

In a further preliminary study of a small group of patients with depressive disorders, we examined pretreatment MHPG excretion as a possible predictor of the clinical antidepressant response to treatment with amitriptyline.[51] As shown in Table XI, sustained antidepressant responses* to treatment with amitriptyline were observed in patients

*A *sustained antidepressant response* was defined as a 50% or greater decrease in Hamilton Depression Rating Scale scores from pretreatment values that was maintained for at least 6 weeks.

TABLE XI. PRETREATMENT MHPG EXCRETION: A POSSIBLE PREDICTOR OF THE ANTIDEPRESSANT RESPONSE TO AMITRIPTYLINE[a]

Patient	Sex	Age	Pretreatment Hamilton Depression Ratings		Pretreatment MHPG excretion[b]		Sustained antidepressant response
			N	Mean	*N*	Mean	
A	F	67	3	42 ± 1	7	3190 ± 230	Yes
B	F	62	4	38 ± 2	7	2240 ± 200	Yes
C	M	55	2	27 ± 1	4	1810 ± 170	Yes
D	F	25	2	29 ± 2	5	1650 ± 80	Yes
E	F	50	2	44 ± 4	3	1590 ± 210	Yes
F	F	44	3	32 ± 2	3	1140 ± 40	No
G	F	18	1	23	2	710 ± 140	No
H	M	28	7	28 ± 2	4	530 ± 80	No

[a]Data reproduced in part from Schildkraut.[51]
[b]Expressed in μg per gram of creatinine.

with relatively higher pretreatment levels of urinary MHPG but not in patients with relatively lower levels. These preliminary findings have recently been confirmed by other investigators.[52]

Conversely, it has been reported that depressed patients who excreted relatively lower levels of MHPG prior to treatment with imipramine or desmethylimipramine responded better to treatment with these antidepressants than did patients who excreted relatively higher levels of MHPG.[9] These findings have been confirmed by one group of investigators[52] but not by another.[8]

On the basis of the initial findings of Maas et al.[9] and Schildkraut,[51] we suggested that the pretreatment levels of MHPG excreted in urine might provide a biochemical criterion for choosing between amitriptyline and imipramine in the treatment of patients with depressive disorders.[51] The recent work of Beckmann and Goodwin[52] provides a preliminary confirmation of this hypothesis.

Our recent neuropharmacological studies have indicated differences as well as similarities in the neurochemical effects of amitriptyline and imipramine or desmethylimipramine.[53–55] Correspondingly, one or another of these tricyclic antidepressants may prove differentially effective in some depressed patients, although clinical experience suggests that other depressed patients may respond to both amitriptyline and imipramine while still others may respond to neither. Thus, our preliminary findings, which will have to be confirmed in more extensive blind studies, suggest that the level of urinary MHPG may provide a clinically useful biochemical criterion for choosing among these tricyclic antidepressants in the treatment of patients with depressive disorders.

CATECHOLAMINES AND CLASSIFICATION OF DEPRESSIONS: PRELIMINARY APPLICATION OF MULTIPLE DISCRIMINANT FUNCTION ANALYSIS

Although in our studies (Tables VIII & X) MHPG was the only catecholamine metabolite that showed a highly significant difference in levels when values in bipolar manic-depressive and unipolar chronic characterological depressions were compared, we could not rule out the possibility that the other urinary metabolites might also contain information which would be useful in differentiating these two types of depressive disorders. In order to explore this possibility, we examined the data obtained from the first 10 patients studied (i.e., 5 bipolar manic-depressive and 5 unipolar chronic characterological depressions) by means of multiple discriminant function analysis. Complete biochemical data were available on a total of 41 urine samples from these patients (i.e., 3 to 6 samples per patient). The biochemical datum from each urine sample was used as a discrete incident (weighting the number of observations from each subject so that all subjects contributed equally to the analysis).* In this analysis, the six catecholamines and metabolites, including norepinephrine, normetanephrine, epinephrine, metanephrine, VMA, and MHPG, as well as various sums and ratios involving the six basic variables, were potential predictors.[57]

A discrimination equation was developed in a "stepwise" procedure where the variable entered into the equation at each step was the one with the largest contribution to discrimination, when the information shared with items already entered was partialed out. This equation was determined by an analytic procedure that obtained the best least squares "fit" of the data and, therefore, was not influenced by the investigators' theoretical framework.

*The heuristic advantages and statistical limitations of such analyses of repeated measures on the same subject (termed *incidence analysis*) are discussed elsewhere.[56]

As shown in Table XII, the equation for "Depression-type" (D-type) score was of the form:

$$\text{D-type score} = C_1(\text{MHPG}) + C_2(\text{VMA}) + C_3(\text{NE}) + C_4 \frac{(\text{NMN}+\text{MN})}{(\text{VMA})} + C_0$$

Each of the four measures selected had a statistically significant contribution to discrimination ($p < .05$), and the overall accuracy of discrimination was highly significant ($p < .001$).* In this formulation, low

*Although this equation was generated mathematically to provide the best least squares fit of the data, one might suggest the following rationale for the terms that were selected:

1. MHPG was the first term to enter the equation as expected from the significant difference in levels observed in bipolar manic-depressive and unipolar chronic characterological depressions. The positive sign of its coefficient indicates that the higher the level of MHPG the more likely the diagnosis of unipolar chronic characterological depression and the less likely the diagnosis of bipolar manic-depressive depression.

2. The inclusion of VMA appears directed to further refining the differentiation between subjects with MHPG levels close to the mean for both groups. In some senses, VMA might be regarded as a "correction" term, perhaps to compensate either for that fraction of urinary MHPG which derives from peripheral sources or for errors in the urine collection procedure. Entering the equation with a minus sign, the level of VMA thus tends to modify the contribution of MHPG. (For example, in the case of a patient with a relatively high VMA as well as a high MHPG, heightened activity of the peripheral sympathetic nervous system might account for a larger fraction of the MHPG than in the case of a patient with a high MHPG but a relatively low VMA. This same reasoning could be applied if one assumed that the VMA might be compensating for inaccuracy in the 24-hour urine collection, since, in the case of a patient with a relatively high VMA as well as a high MHPG, the urine collection could conceivably have extended beyond the normal 24-hour period resulting in a general increase in the levels of all metabolites, whereas in the case of a patient with relatively low VMA but high MHPG one could not simply ascribe the elevation of MHPG to an excessively long period of urine collection.)

3. Norepinephrine may be introduced into the equation with a positive coefficient on the basis of the tendency for bipolar manic-depressives to have relatively lower levels of urinary norepinephrine than patients with unipolar chronic characterological depressions.

4. The ratio (normetanephrine + metanephrine) : VMA enters the equation with a negative coefficient, indicating that the higher this ratio the more likely that a patient is bipolar manic-depressive. This ratio may correspond to the N/O ratio of urinary amines to deaminated metabolites of intravenously administered radioactive norepinephrine, which Rosenblatt and Chanley[58] have found to be higher in patients with retarded depressions classified as manic-depressives than in patients with other types of depressions. The (NMN+MN) : VMA ratio (as well as Rosenblatt and Chanley's N/O ratio), moreover, may be reflecting differences in monoamine oxidase activity between these types of depressive disorders. Since normetanephrine and metanephrine can be converted to VMA (or MHPG) by deamination, this ratio may be inversely related to monoamine oxidase activity. As noted above, on the basis of measurements of platelet monoamine oxidase activity, other investigators[49] have suggested that monoamine oxidase activity may be relatively reduced in patients with bipolar manic-depressive disorders; and this would be consistent with the fact that the ratio (normetanephrine + metanephrine) : VMA enters the equation with a negative coefficient.

TABLE XII. DISCRIMINATION EQUATION FOR D-TYPE SCORE

$$\text{D-type score} = C_1(\text{MHPG}) + C_2(\text{VMA}) + C_3(\text{NE}) + C_4\frac{(\text{NMN} + \text{MN})}{(\text{VMA})} + C_o$$

Coefficients and constant	Standardized coefficients
$C_1 = 3.734 \times 10^{-4}$	0.438
$C_2 = -2.303 \times 10^{-4}$	−0.454
$C_3 = 1.035 \times 10^{-2}$	0.420
$C_4 = -4.217$	−0.389
$C_o = 0.918$	—

scores (< 0.5) are related to bipolar manic-depressive depressions and high scores (> 0.5) are related to unipolar chronic characterological depressions.

Preliminary validation of this discrimination equation has been obtained in a sample of 25 additional depressed patients whose biochemical data had not been used to derive the equation. In this validation sample, all of the patients with schizoaffective or bipolar manic-depressive depressions had D-type scores below 0.500 (in fact the largest D-type score in this subgroup was 0.381), while all of the patients with unipolar chronic characterological or unipolar nonspecific depressions had D-type scores above 0.500 (Table XIII and Figure 4).

In addition to the patients with schizoaffective or bipolar manic-depressive depressions, 3 of the 8 patients with unipolar endogenous depressions also had D-type scores below 0.500 (Table XIII). Such

TABLE XIII. D-TYPE SCORES[a] IN DEPRESSIVE DISORDERS: PRELIMINARY VALIDATION SAMPLE

D-type scores	Bipolar manic-depressive and schizoaffective	Unipolar endogenous	Unipolar chronic characterological and nonspecific
Mean ± SEM	0.237 ± 0.032	0.545 ± 0.089	0.651 ± 0.033
Range	0.142 to 0.381	0.252 to 0.942	0.534 to 0.757
	(N = 9)	(N = 8)	(N = 8)

[a]D-type scores were computed using the biochemical data from 2 to 6 separate 24-hour urine samples obtained from each patient. The average D-type score for each patient was used to compute the group means ± standard errors of the means presented in this table. N = number of patients.

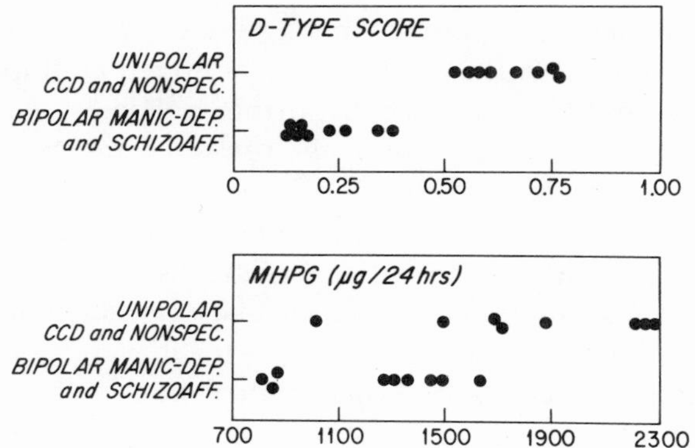

Figure 4. D-type scores and MHPG excretion in depressed patients: preliminary validation ($N=17$). Individual values of the D-type scores and MHPG excretion are plotted for the group of schizoaffective or bipolar manic-depressive depressions and the group of unipolar chronic characterological (CCD) or nonspecific depressions in the preliminary validation sample.

D-type scores below 0.500 may conceivably help to identify, from within the group of unipolar endogenous depressions, those patients with a biochemical similarity or predisposition to bipolar manic-depressive (or schizoaffective) disorders even though the patient may not have had overt episodes of hypomania or mania (or other forms of excited states).

This possibility is illustrated by the case of a 60-year-old man who was studied biochemically during his fourth endogenous depressive episode. Since he had never had a prior episode of hypomania or mania, at the time of the biochemical studies, he was considered to have a unipolar endogenous depressive disorder. However, his D-type score (0.381) was in the range usually seen in schizoaffective or bipolar manic-depressive depressions. One year after the biochemical studies were performed, this patient experienced his first hypomanic episode. Thus, it is possible that the D-type score may be of use in identifying depressed patients with a latent predisposition to bipolar manic-depressive illness prior to the appearance of the first overt manic or hypomanic episode.

Figure 4, which compares individual values of the D-type scores and MHPG excretion in the group of schizoaffective or bipolar manic-depressive depressions and the group of unipolar chronic characterological or nonspecific depressions in the preliminary validation sample, shows that there was no overlap and a very wide separation of the

D-type scores in these two groups, whereas there was some overlap and less separation of the MHPG levels. Thus, although additional studies using a larger sample are needed to further validate and refine this equation for obtaining D-type scores, the present findings suggest that this equation may provide an even more precise discrimination between these types of depressive disorders than does urinary MHPG alone. In this regard, it is intriguing to speculate that the discrimination equation, by including the contribution of various urinary catecholamine metabolites of peripheral origin, may be correcting for that fraction of urinary MHPG that derives from the periphery rather than the brain.

PRELIMINARY STUDIES OF THE USE OF PLATELET MONOAMINE OXIDASE ACTIVITY IN CONJUNCTION WITH MHPG EXCRETION AS A FURTHER CRITERION FOR CLASSIFYING DEPRESSIVE DISORDERS

We have recently begun to examine platelet monoamine oxidase activity in conjunction with MHPG and other urinary catecholamine metabolites in our studies of patients with depressive disorders. Up to the present time we have analyzed data on 25 patients, some of whom were included in previous studies. However, in this phase of our research we included a broader range of clinical diagnostic entities inasmuch as we did not exclude patients with histories of chronic asocial, eccentric, or bizarre behavior, patients with histories of prior amphetamine or barbiturate abuse, or patients with depressions that could not be uniquely classified according to our system of classification.[34]

Preliminary findings suggest that the measurement of platelet monoamine oxidase activity (using tryptamine as substrate) may enable us to make clinically relevant distinctions within the group of depressed patients with relatively low MHPG excretion (i.e., less than 1500 μg/day). The study of Murphy and Weiss[49] reporting low platelet monoamine oxidase activity in bipolar affective disorders, in conjunction with our findings of relatively low MHPG excretion in depressed patients with bipolar manic-depressive disorders, suggests that there should be a subgroup of depressive disorders with low MHPG excretion and low platelet monoamine oxidase activity that includes bipolar manic-depressive depressions as well as other biologically related disorders; and our preliminary findings support this possibility. However, as shown in Table

TABLE XIV. CHRONIC ASOCIAL BEHAVIOR AND PSYCHOTIC DISORGANIZATION ON TRICYCLIC ANTIDEPRESSANTS IN DEPRESSED PATIENTS WITH LOW MHPG EXCRETION AND HIGH PLATELET MAO ACTIVITY

	Chronic asocial behavior[a,b]	Psychotic disorganization on tricyclic antidepressants[b]
MHPG < 1500[c]		
MAO > 7.0[d]	5/6	4/6
MAO <7.0	0/7	1/7
MHPG > 1500		
MAO > 7.0	2/6	0/6
MAO < 7.0	0/6	0/6

[a]Chronic asocial behavior includes deterioration in functioning, extreme social isolation, or odd, bizarre, eccentric behavior of at least several years duration.
[b]Fraction of patients showing this manifestation.
[c]MHPG excretion is expressed in μg/24 hours.
[d]Platelet monoamine oxidase (MAO) activity is expressed in nanomoles of tryptamine deaminated/hour/milligram of platelet protein.

XIV, our data further suggest that the occurrence of relatively high platelet monoamine oxidase activity (i.e., greater than 7 nmol tryptamine deaminated/hr/mg protein) in conjunction with low MHPG excretion (less than 1500 μg/day) may help to discriminate a further subgroup of depressive disorders, characterized clinically by histories of chronic asocial, eccentric, or bizarre behavior and by the propensity for psychotic disorganization (clinically distinguishable from hypomanic or manic states) particularly when treated with tricyclic antidepressant drugs.

As shown in Table XIV, 5 of the 6 patients with urinary MHPG less than 1500 μg/day and platelet monoamine oxidase activity greater than 7 nmol tryptamine deaminated/hr/mg protein had histories of chronic asocial, eccentric, or bizarre behavior, and 4 of these 6 patients (including the one without chronic asocial behavior) had experienced psychotic disorganization when treated with tricyclic antidepressant drugs. In contrast, none of the 7 patients with low MHPG excretion and low platelet MAO activity had histories of chronic asocial, eccentric, or bizarre behavior, and only 1 of these 7 patients had a history of psychotic disorganization on tricyclic antidepressants. Of the remaining 12 subjects (i.e., with MHPG greater than 1500 μg/day) only 2 had histories of chronic asocial, eccentric, or bizarre behavior, and none manifested psychosis during treatment with tricyclic antidepressants (Table XIV).

The patients in the subgroup with relatively low MHPG excretion and relatively high platelet monoamine oxidase activity had frequently received clinical diagnoses (at other facilities) in the schizophrenia spectrum including schizophrenia and schizoid or schizoaffective disorders, and the term *borderline* was sometimes used to describe them. It should be emphasized, however, that our research classification of *schizoaffective disorders* does not include patients with histories of chronic asocial, eccentric, or bizarre behavior,[34]* and such patients were not included among the *schizoaffective disorders* that we grouped with bipolar manic-depressive disorders in our studies demonstrating low D-type scores in these disorders (Table XIII). Further analyses are in progress to determine D-type scores in the group of patients with low MHPG excretion and high platelet MAO activity, but preliminary data on 4 patients suggest they may not have low D-type scores.

Thus, our preliminary findings suggest that depressed patients with relatively low MHPG excretion and relatively high platelet monoamine oxidase activity may constitute a biochemically identifiable and clinically relevant subgroup of depressive disorders that includes patients with histories of chronic asocial, eccentric, or bizarre behavior and with a propensity for psychotic disorganization particularly when treated with tricyclic antidepressants. In contrast, depressed patients with low MHPG excretion and relatively low platelet monoamine oxidase activity may constitute another subgroup of depressive disorders that includes bipolar manic-depressive and related disorders. Further studies will clearly be required to confirm these very preliminary findings.

CONCLUSION

In summary, we have observed that MHPG excretion was higher during hypomanias or manias, intermediate during well intervals, and

*According to our research classification, depressive disorders with histories of chronic asocial behavior (which includes deterioration in functioning, extreme social isolation or odd, bizarre, eccentric behavior of at least several years' duration) plus evidence of a well-documented schizophrenic psychosis, characterized by thought disorders and delusions or hallucinations that are not affect consonant, are termed *true schizophrenia-related depressive disorders*. Depressive disorders with histories of chronic asocial behavior but without evidence of overt psychosis are termed *schizoid-affective disorders*. As we use it, the term *schizoaffective disorder* is restricted to depressive or manic disorders without histories of chronic asocial behavior but with histories of psychotic manifestations (including transient micropsychotic episodes) that are not solely affect consonant.

lower during depressions in longitudinal studies of patients with bipolar manic-depressive disorders. In cross-sectional comparisons of groups of patients with various clinically defined subtypes of depressive disorders, examined prior to treatment with antidepressant drugs or electroconvulsive therapy, we have observed that MHPG excretion was significantly lower in patients with schizoaffective or bipolar manic-depressive depressions than in patients with unipolar chronic characterological or unipolar nonspecific depressions. Extending these findings, our studies (using multiple discriminant function analysis) suggest that an equation which includes other measures related to catecholamine metabolism in addition to MHPG may provide a more precise discrimination among these subtypes of depressive disorders than does urinary MHPG alone.

Moreover, recent preliminary findings suggest that the measurement of platelet monoamine oxidase activity may enable us to make clinically relevant distinctions within the group of depressed patients with relatively low MHPG excretion. Our findings, together with those of other investigators, suggest that there is a subgroup of depressive disorders with low MHPG excretion and low platelet monoamine oxidase activity that includes bipolar manic-depressive depressions as well as other biologically related disorders. However, our recent preliminary findings also suggest that another subgroup of depressive disorders, characterized clinically by chronic asocial, eccentric, or bizarre behavior and by a propensity for psychotic disorganization particularly on tricyclic antidepressants, may be discriminated on the basis of relatively high platelet monoamine oxidase activity occurring in conjunction with relatively low MHPG excretion.

In the aggregate, these findings provide further evidence that alterations in central norepinephrine metabolism may be of importance in the underlying pathophysiology of at least some types of depressive disorders, and these findings also suggest that various measures related to catecholamine metabolism may provide a clinically useful biochemical basis for classifying the depressive disorders. While further studies will be required to confirm this, the present findings do provide support for the possibility, suggested a number of years ago,[3] that biochemical measures related to catecholamine metabolism may help to differentiate among the subtypes of depressive disorders.

It must be stressed, however, that alterations in other biochemical systems, including the indoleamines, also have been observed in depressed patients, and there is evidence that these biochemical factors also may be of value in classifying the depressive disorders.[2] Since it is generally agreed that clinically defined diagnostic groupings of depressions do not necessarily represent biologically homogeneous entities, the use of biochemical criteria in conjunction with specific clinical criteria could conceivably lead to new diagnostic categories that are biologically more meaningful and therapeutically more relevant than those defined by clinical criteria alone. Indeed, one can foresee the possibility of biochemical tests soon being used as routinely in the diagnostic workup of patients with depressive disorders as they are now in the evaluation of patients with endocrinopathies or other types of metabolic disorders.

ACKNOWLEDGMENTS

This work was supported in part by USPHS Grant No. MH-15413 and by a grant from the Scottish Rite Schizophrenia Research Program, N.M.J., U.S.A.

The authors wish to thank Mr. Edwin Grab, Ms. Patricia Platz, Ms. Sandra Lipchus, Mr. Vincent DaForno, and Ms. Barbara Keeler for their technical assistance.

REFERENCES

1. Schildkraut JJ: *Neuropsychopharmacology and the Affective Disorders.* Boston, Little, Brown, 1970.
2. Schildkraut JJ: Biogenic amines and affective disorders. *Ann. Rev. Med. 25:*333–348, 1974.
3. Schildkraut JJ: The catecholamine hypothesis of affective disorders: A review of supporting evidence. *Am. J. Psychiatry 122:*509–522, 1965.
4. Axelrod J: Noradrenaline: Fate and control of its biosynthesis. *Science 173:*598–606, 1971.
5. Kopin IJ, Gordon EK: Metabolism of norepinephrine-H^3 released by tyramine and reserpine. *J. Pharmacol. Exp. Ther. 138:*351–359, 1962.
6. Kopin IJ, Gordon EK: Metabolism of administered and drug-released norepinephrine-7-H^3 in rat. *J. Pharmacol. Exp. Ther. 140:*207–219, 1963.
7. Schildkraut JJ, Green R, Gordon EK, Durell J: Normetanephrine excretion and affective state in depressed patients treated with imipramine. *Am. J. Psychiatry 123:*690–700, 1966.
8. Prange AJ Jr., Wilson IC, Knox AE, McClane TK, Breese GR, Martin BR, Alltop LB, Lipton MA: Thyroid-imipramine clinical and chemical interaction: Evidence for a receptor deficit in depression. *J. Psychiat. Res. 9:*187–206, 1972.

9. Maas JW, Fawcett JA, Dekirmenjian H: Catecholamine metabolism, depressive illness and drug response. *Arch. Gen. Psychiatry 26:*252–262, 1972.
10. Weil-Malherbe H, Axelrod J, Tomchick R: Blood–brain barrier for adrenaline. *Science 129:*1226–1227, 1959.
11. Glowinski J, Kopin IJ, Axelrod J: Metabolism of (H^3) norepinephrine in rat brain. *J. Neurochem. 12:*25–30, 1965.
12. Schanberg SM, Schildkraut JJ, Breese GR, Kopin IJ: Metabolism of normetanephrine-H^3 in rat brain—Identification of conjugated 3-methoxy-4-hydroxy-phenylglycol as major metabolite. *Biochem. Pharmacol. 17:*247–254, 1968.
13. Schanberg SM, Breese GR, Schildkraut JJ, Gordon EK, Kopin IJ: 3-Methoxy-4-hydroxyphenylglycol sulfate in brain and cerebrospinal fluid. *Biochem. Pharmacol. 17:*2006–2008, 1968.
14. Maas JW, Landis DH: *In vivo* studies of metabolism of norepinephrine in central nervous system. *J. Pharmacol. Exp. Ther. 163:*147–162, 1968.
15. Maas JW, Fawcett JA, Dekirmenjian H: 3-Methoxy-4-hydroxyphenylglycol (MHPG) excretion in depressive states: Pilot study. *Arch. Gen. Psychiatry 19:*129–134, 1968.
16. Mannarino E, Kirshner N, Nashold BS Jr: Metabolism of C^{14} noradrenaline by cat brain *in vivo. J. Neurochem. 10:*373–379, 1963.
17. Rutledge CO, Jonason J: Metabolic pathways of dopamine and norepinephrine in rabbit brain *in vitro. J. Pharmacol. Exp. Ther. 157:*493–502, 1967.
18. Wilk S, Watson E: VMA in spinal fluid: Evaluation of the pathways of cerebral catecholamine metabolism in man. In: Usdin E, Snyder S (eds) *Frontiers In Catecholamine Research—Third International Catecholamine Symposium,* pp. 1067–1069. New York, Pergamon, 1973.
19. Chase TN, Breese GR, Gordon EK, Kopin IJ: Catecholamine metabolism in the dog: Comparison of intravenously and intraventricularly administered (^{14}C) dopamine and (^3H) norepinephrine. *J. Neurochem. 18:*135–140, 1971.
20. Axelrod J, Kopin IJ, Mann JD: 3-Methoxy-4-hydroxyphenylglycol sulfate, a new metabolite of epinephrine and norepinephrine. *Biochim. Biophys. Acta 36:*576–577, 1959.
21. Maas JW, Dekirmenjian H, Garver D, Redmond DE Jr., Landis DH: Catecholamine metabolite excretion following intraventricular injection of 60H-dopamine. *Brain Res. 41:*507–511, 1972.
22. Breese GR, Prange AJ Jr, Howard JL, Lipton MA, McKinney WT, Bowman RE, Bushnell P: 3-Methoxy-4-hydroxyphenylglycol excretion and behavioral changes in rat and monkey after central sympathectomy with 6-hydroxy-dopamine. *Nature New Biol. 240:*286–87, 1972.
23. Kopin I, Ebert M: Recent preliminary studies of the metabolism of catecholamines in the periphery and brain of human subjects. Reported at the Symposium on The Biological Deficit in the Affective Disorders, Munich, Germany, October 1974.
24. Greenspan K, Schildkraut JJ, Gordon EK, Baer L, Aranoff MS, Durell J: Catecholamine metabolism in affective disorders III. MHPG and other catecholamine metabolites in patients treated with lithium carbonate. *J. Psychiat. Res. 7:*171–183, 1970.
25. Schildkraut JJ, Keeler BA, Rogers MP, Draskoczy PR: Catecholamine metabolism in affective disorders: A longitudinal study of a patient treated with amitriptyline and ECT. *Psychosom. Med. 34:*470, 1972; plus erratum: *Psychosom. Med. 35:*274, 1973.
26. Schildkraut JJ, Watson R, Draskoczy PR, Hartmann E: Amphetamine withdrawal: Depression and MHPG excretion. *Lancet ii:*485–486, 1971.
27. Watson R, Hartmann E, Schildkraut JJ: Amphetamine withdrawal: Affective state, sleep patterns and MHPG excretion. *Am. J. Psychiatry 129:*263–269, 1972.

28. Bond PA, Jenner FA, Sampson GA: Daily variations of the urine content of 3-methoxy-4-hydroxyphenylglycol in two manic-depressive patients. *Psychol. Med. 2:*81–85, 1972.
29. Jones FD, Maas JW, Dekirmenjian H, Fawcett JA: Urinary catecholamine metabolites during behavioral changes in a patient with manic-depressive cycles. *Science 179:*300–302, 1973.
30. Bunney WE Jr, Goodwin FK, Murphy DL, House KM, Gordon EK: The "switch process" in manic-depressive illness. *Arch. Gen. Psychiatry 27:*304–309, 1972.
31. Shopsin B, Wilk W, Gershon S, Roffman M, Goldstein M: Collaborative psychopharmacologic studies exploring catecholamine metabolism in psychiatric disorders. In: Usdin E, Snyder S (eds) *Frontiers in Catecholamine Research—Third International Catecholamine Symposium,* pp. 1173–1179. New York, Pergamon, 1973.
32. Schildkraut JJ, Keeler BA, Papousek M, Hartmann E: MHPG excretion in depressive disorders: Relation to clinical subtypes and desynchronized sleep. *Science 181:*762–764, 1973.
33. Schildkraut JJ, Keeler BA, Grab EL, Kantrowich J, Hartmann E: MHPG excretion and clinical classification in depressive disorders. *Lancet i:*1251–1252, 1973.
34. Schildkraut JJ, Klein DF: The classification and treatment of depressive disorders. In: Shader RI (ed) *Manual of Psychiatric Therapeutics,* pp. 39–61. Boston, Little, Brown, 1975.
35. Ebert MH, Post RM, Goodwin FK: Effect of physical activity on urinary MHPG excretion in depressed patients. *Lancet ii:*766, 1972.
36. Maas JW, Dekirmenjian H, Fawcett J: Catecholamine metabolism, depression and stress. *Nature 230:*330–331, 1971.
37. Rubin RT, Miller RG, Clark BR, Poland RE, Arthur RJ: The stress of aircraft carrier landings II. 3-Methoxy-4-hydroxyphenylglycol excretion in naval aviators. *Psychosom. Med. 32:*589–597, 1970.
38. Hamilton M: A rating scale for depression. *J. Neurol. Neurosurg. Psychiatry 23:*56–62, 1960.
39. Schildkraut JJ: Catecholamine metabolism and affective disorders: Studies of MHPG excretion. In: Usdin E, Snyder S (eds) *Frontiers In Catecholamine Research—Third International Catecholamine Symposium,* pp. 1165–1171. New York, Pergamon, 1973.
40. Maas JW, Dekirmenjian H, Jones F: The identification of depressed patients who have a disorder of norepinephrine metabolism and/or disposition. In: Usdin E, Snyder S (eds) *Frontiers in Catecholamine Research—Third International Catecholamine Symposium,* pp. 1091–1096. New York, Pergamon, 1973.
41. Schildkraut JJ: Mania-depression rating scale, unpublished, 1961.
42. Hartmann E: Longitudinal studies of sleep and dream patterns in manic-depressive patients. *Arch. Gen. Psychiatry 19:*312–329, 1968.
43. Detre T, Himmelhoch J, Swartzburg M, Anderson CM, Byck R, Kupfer DJ: Hypersomnia and manic-depressive disease. *Am. J. Psychiatry 128:*1303–1305, 1972.
44. Kupfer DJ, Himmelhoch JM, Swartzburg M, Anderson C, Byck R, Detre TP: Hypersomnia in manic-depressive disease. *Dis. Nerv. Syst. 33:*720–724, 1972.
45. Goodwin FK, Beckmann H, Post RM: Urinary methoxy-4-hydroxyphenylglycol in subtypes of affective illness. *Scientific Proceedings,* Annual Meeting, American Psychiatric Association, pp. 96–97, 1975.
46. Jones FD, Maas JW, Dekirmenjian H, Sanchez J: Diagnostic subtypes of affective disorders and their urinary excretion of catecholamine metabolites. *Am. J. Psychiatry 132:*1141–1148, 1975.
47. Murphy DL, Wyatt RJ: Reduced monoamine oxidase activity in blood platelets from schizophrenic patients. *Nature 238:*225–226, 1972.

48. Schildkraut JJ, Herzog JM, Orsulak PJ, Edelman SE, Shein HM, Frazier SH: Reduced platelet monoamine oxidase activity in a subgroup of schizophrenic patients. *Am. J. Psychiatry 133:*438–440, 1976.
49. Murphy DL, Weiss R: Reduced monoamine oxidase activity in blood platelets from bipolar depressed patients. *Am. J. Psychiatry 128:*1351–1357, 1972.
50. Nies A, Robinson DS, Ravaris CL, Davis JM: Amines and monoamine oxidase in relation to aging and depression in man. *Psychosom. Med. 33:*470, 1971.
51. Schildkraut JJ: Norepinephrine metabolites as biochemical criteria for classifying depressive disorders and predicting responses to treatment: Preliminary findings. *Am. J. Psychiatry 130:*695–699, 1973.
52. Beckmann H, Goodwin FK: Antidepressant response to tricyclics and urinary MHPG in unipolar patients: Clinical response to imipramine or amitriptyline. *Arch. Gen. Psychiatry 32:*17–21, 1975.
53. Schildkraut JJ, Dodge GA, Logue MA: Effects of tricyclic antidepressants on the uptake and metabolism of intracisternally administered norepinephrine-H^3 in rat brain. *J. Psychiat. Res. 7:*29–34, 1969.
54. Schildkraut JJ, Draskoczy PR, Gershon ES, Reich P, Grab EL: Effects of tricyclic antidepressants on norepinephrine metabolism: Basic and clinical studies. In: Ho BT, McIsaac WM (eds) *Brain Chemistry and Mental Disease,* pp. 215–236. New York, Plenum, 1971.
55. Schildkraut JJ, Draskoczy PR, Gershon ES, Reich P, Grab EL: Catecholamine metabolism in affective disorders IV. Preliminary studies of norepinephrine metabolism in depressed patients treated with amitriptyline. *J. Psychiat. Res. 9:*173–185, 1972.
56. LaBrie RA: Incidence analyses, unpublished.
57. Schildkraut JJ, LaBrie RA: Catecholamines and classification of depressions. *New Research Abstracts,* American Psychiatric Association Annual Meeting, p. 17, 1974.
58. Rosenblatt S, Chanley JD: Differences in metabolism of norpinephrine in depressions: Effects of various therapies. *Arch. Gen. Psychiatry 13:*495–502, 1965.

4

The Amine Hypothesis Revisited: A Clinician's View

LEO E. HOLLISTER

It is worth remembering the simple syllogism which led to the amine hypothesis of depression. A number of workers, including myself, had shown in 1954 that reserpine would produce depression, even in nondepressed normal subjects. Subsequent pharmacologic studies of its mode of action showed that it impaired the storage in nerve endings of serotonin, of norepinephrine, and, ultimately, of dopamine. Thus, the conclusion was reached that depression was associated with a depletion of neurotransmission due to one or the other of these amines. In some parts of the world norepinephrine was favored, while in others it was serotonin; the role of dopamine is still unclear.

Studies of antidepressant drugs, however, confirmed the diversity of depressions which had long been recognized by a confusing array of diagnostic terms. Only depressions which might be classified as "endogenous" showed a clear response to drugs. Thus the amine hypotheses of depression were limited to this category, as opposed to "reactive" depressions. The latter were believed to be due to life experiences and amenable to treatment of psychosocial means, while the former were believed to represent a biological interaction in a person vulnerable to depression due to a genetic–biochemical abnormality and best treated by pharmacologic means.

The conflict over which amines were important in endogenous depressions has never been resolved, but with evidence mounting that both might be involved, some attempts to reconciliation were attempted. Serotonin was alleged to set the affective tone—that is, its diminished transmission would make one depressed—while norepine-

LEO E. HOLLISTER • Department of Psychiatry, Stanford University School of Medicine, Palo Alto, California.

phrine set the behavioral consequences, too little noradrenergic transmission being associated with a "retarded" depression and too much with an "agitated" depression. Later, this concept was extended to explain manic-depressive disorder, with too little catecholaminergic transmission being associated with depression and too much with mania.

That manic-depressive disorder should be confused with endogenous depression is more likely clinically than it should be on any theoretical basis. Available evidence suggests that it is truly a different entity with a separate type of genetic transmission and quite possibly a different biochemical mechanism. Its response is greatest to lithium rather than to the antidepressant drugs, although the latter may be useful in the depressed phase. To make matters more confusing, the terms *unipolar* and *bipolar* have been introduced, based on the assumption that mania and depression are poles of a continuum in which *normal* is in the middle, an assumption which is completely unproven. Unipolar and bipolar depression have been further subdivided, increasing the confusion in much of the current literature. The only consistent part of this unfortunate nomenclature is that *bipolar* usually refers to some variant of manic-depressive disorder.

THE AMINE HYPOTHESIS REVISITED

The amine hypothesis of depression was singularly attractive, for it promised simultaneously to explain the biochemical pathogenesis of depression and the mode of action of antidepressant drugs. One of the earliest methods for studying the amine hypothesis was to measure the urinary excretion of norepinephrine or serotonin and their metabolites. After a prodigious amount of work had been done, it became clear that these measurements were a laborious and expensive way to process sewage. The wrong things had been measured. The important urinary metabolite of norepinephrine was found to be 3-methoxy-4-hydroxyphenylglycol (MHPG), which may represent variable amounts of norepinephrine activity in the brain. In the case of serotonin, measurement of the accumulation of its metabolite, 5-hydroxyindoleacetic acid (5HIAA), in cerebrospinal fluid rather than in the urine was a more accurate indicator of its activity in the brain. Such measurements had to be done with probenecid block of the egress of the metabolite from the fluid, a somewhat cumbersome procedure. Thus, what seemed at first to be a simple hypothesis, the testing of which might be accomplished with relatively simple (in retrospect) methods, no longer was the case.

The simple amine hypothesis was especially reassuring when the mechanism of action of tricyclic antidepressants was considered. Although they have sedative, central antimuscarinic, and amine-pump blocking actions, it is the latter which is deemed crucial to their therapeutic effect in endogenous depressions. A possible reason why some patients failed to respond to adequate treatment with a tricyclic was that the wrong drug was chosen for their specific type of neurotransmitter disorder. Tertiary amines had been found to block selectively uptake of serotonin, while secondary amines preferentially blocked norepinephrine uptake. This interesting pharmacologic difference between tricyclics has never yet been adequately tested in the clinic, due in some part to the great difficulty in making such clear biochemical distinctions and to the fact that tertiary amines are, to varying extents, metabolized to secondary amines.

Matters were made more complicated by the observation that (a) the simple deficiency-of-amine-transmission hypothesis may not be true—depressions could be categorized on a bimodal distribution based on either low or high urinary excretion of the major CNS metabolite of norepinephrine, MHPG; and (b) imipramine was specifically effective in patients with low MHPG excretion and the converse was true for amitriptyline. Thus, not only were there differences between secondary and tertiary amine tricyclics but even between the tertiary amines.

Until the reports of the differences between the tertiary amines, it had been virtually impossible to make any distinctions between them in terms of their overall clinical efficacy, other than that both were more effective treatments than placebo when applied to patients clearly diagnosed as having endogenous depression. If the rule found with excretion of norepinephrine metabolites holds for other neurotransmitters, we might conceivably have four to six biochemical types of depression, based on either increased or decreased excretion of metabolites of norepinephrine, serotonin, or dopamine.

The discovery that all endogenous depression was not associated with a decreased excretion of a neurotransmitter metabolite but that the distribution was bimodally low or high was one of several lines of evidence that have led to a reexamination of the amine hypothesis of depression. Recent evidence from the study of CSF metabolites of serotonin suggests that with this neurotransmitter a bimodal distribution of serotonin turnover is found in depression. To confuse matters further both tricyclics of the tertiary amine type reduce serotonin turnover still further. Finally, all the available evidence indicates that increasing brain concentrations of serotonin are associated with sedation, which simply may reflect the greater sedative action of tertiary amine tricyclics.

The importance of the amine pump mechanism is being questioned by exceptions to the rule provided by doxepin (a weak drug in this respect) and iprindole, which is inactive; both are reported to be effective clinically. Further, although block of the amine pump is immediate, clinical response is usually delayed.

Attempts to treat depression by giving precursors of neurotransmitters have not been generally successful. Neither *l*-tryptophan nor 1,5-hydroxytryptophan can be considered as of proven value. Levodopa aggravates rather than helps most depressions, but it increases only dopamine, not norepinephrine. An adequate clinical trial of a precursor of norepinephrine has not been done. Inhibition of synthesizing enzymes, by means of parachlorphenylalamine (PCPA) for serotonin, or alpha-methylparatyrosine (AMPT) for norepinephrine, has not aggravated depression. The inhibition for catabolizing enzymes by monoamine oxidase inhibitors has generally been less successful in treating depression than other approaches, and therapeutic action could be due to other pharmacologic effects.

THE CONFUSED CLINICIAN

What should the clinician now do? First, he should continue, as best he can, to make diagnostic distinctions between the major affective disorders. Second, endogenous depressions should be treated with tricyclic drugs given in adequate doses (probably assured by measuring plasma concentrations) for reasonably long periods. One may or may not wish to supplant the same tertiary amine tricyclic with equivalent amounts of its secondary amine metabolite to see if response can be improved in patients who respond poorly. In desperate cases, one may wish to try the same procedures with the other tertiary amine. Third, until much better methods are worked out for routine measurement of urinary and CSF metabolites of neurotransmitters, the average clinician should not feel obliged to try to obtain such measurements on his patients.

5

Why We Do Not Yet Understand the Genetics of Affective Disorders

KENNETH K. KIDD and MYRNA M. WEISSMAN

INTRODUCTION

Reasonably good evidence exists for at least some types of affective disorders having a genetic component. Consequently, there are many recent reviews of the data supporting genetic hypotheses for the affective disorders.[1–4] Since no remarkable new evidence has appeared in the last couple of years, those reviews still provide good summaries of the data. However, considerable debate occurs over the interpretation of these data, and new thoughts are developing in this area. In this chapter we shall briefly review the evidence needed for determining whether a genetic component exists, discuss the current data and analyses relative to mode(s) of inheritance for affective disorders, and finally discuss the types of data that are still required in order to resolve the uncertainties. The absence of these types of data and the difficulty in obtaining them explain, as we shall show, why we do not yet understand the genetics of affective disorders.

Evidence Needed for a Genetic Hypothesis

The genetic element of a disease is obvious if an enzyme or structural protein is altered or absent. Certain other biochemical aberrations are presumptive evidence of genetic defects even in the absence of family data. However, for the affective disorders, biochemical studies have not yet provided evidence for any genetic defect. Four other types of

KENNETH K. KIDD and MYRNA M. WEISSMAN • Department of Human Genetics, Yale University School of Medicine, New Haven, Connecticut; Depression Research Unit, Connecticut Mental Health Center, Department of Psychiatry, Yale University School of Medicine, New Haven, Connecticut.

evidence can suggest that genetic factors are responsible for a disease of unknown etiology: (a) a higher concordance among monozygotic (MZ) twins than among dizygotic (DZ) twins; (b) significant aggregation of the illness within families; (c) genetic linkage of the illness with an identifiable allele at a marker locus; (d) a higher incidence of the trait, irrespective of home environment, among biological offspring of affected individuals than among biological offspring of unaffected individuals, i.e., a "positive" adoption study. Twin studies and studies of biological families are incapable of proving the existence of genetic factors for traits that might have a major environmental component in their etiology because genes and environment are confounded in determining similarities among relatives and cannot be separately quantified. Although genetic linkage and adoption studies can demonstrate that genetic factors must be important, such studies are difficult to conduct and are not commonly done. Even when done they can still give ambiguous results.

In the absence of a well-understood etiology, demonstration of the presence of genetic factors does not usually resolve questions about the nature of the genes involved and how they interact with environmental factors. Is a particular gene necessary for the disease to develop? Will a certain genotype always lead to illness? Are there ameliorating environments that prevent illness in persons otherwise susceptible? Answers to questions such as these usually require data of many different types. The full scope of genetic–environment interactions can only be understood after the full disease process is understood. Until such a time, family data—pedigrees—and data on genetic linkage can be the bases for an initial understanding.

For affective disorders, the evidence from twin studies, family studies, and genetic linkage studies is consistent with a major genetic contribution. No nontwin adoption studies have been reported, though an important one is under way in Scandinavia. While it does seem likely that genetic factors are indeed present, considerable uncertainty remains about the mode(s) of inheritance of the affective disorders.

Accurate Diagnosis and Population Rates

Two other considerations are vital for the interpretation of all evidence relative to genetic factors: (a) accurate definition of the trait, i.e., diagnosis, and (b) knowledge of the chance that a random individual will be affected, i.e., the population incidence. Deficits in both these areas, as will be described, have hindered research on the genetics of affective disorders.

Diagnosis. Genetic studies of affective disorders whether twin, family, linkage, or adoption studies have until recently been hampered by the imprecision and variability in diagnostic criteria. In fact, most variation in results among different studies can be explained by the differences in diagnostic methods. There are two major sources of unreliability in diagnosis: first in the method of collecting information necessary for making diagnostic distinctions and second in the rules for using the data to classify patients into diagnostic categories. New diagnostic methodologies which take into account these sources of variation and improve reliability considerably have become available[5] and are now being applied to genetic studies. Other recent developments in psychopathology that are relevant to diagnosis include efforts to standardize cross-cultural differences in diagnosis[6,7] and to develop and utilize approaches to validating diagnosis.[8]

Greater diagnostic differentiation is now standard, particularly the separation of affective disorders into two groups[9]—unipolar (UP) and bipolar (BP). *Unipolar* includes persons with a major depressive illness only, usually of a recurring nature (although that aspect of the definition varies), and *bipolar* includes persons with episodes of both mania and depression. These two groups have been shown to differ in several ways; e.g., bipolars have an earlier age of onset (median about 26 years) than unipolars (median about 40 years). Subsequent genetic, psychopharmacologic, and clinical studies support this distinction. The newest methods of diagnosis make the bipolar–unipolar distinction and also include milder forms of bipolar and several forms of unipolar disorders. The improved definition of diagnostic categories and the greater accuracy with which patients can be classified will undoubtedly improve future genetic studies.

Population Incidence. The absence of comparable population incidence data in the United States has been a major difficulty in interpreting the available family data. Much of the population data considered in genetic studies derives from rates of treated cases. Clinical data of treated patients are insufficient for several reasons: the treated samples are not representative of all persons with the disorder, ascertainment is incomplete, the more serious forms of illness are overrepresented, and diagnostic criteria are uncontrolled.

Accurate estimation of the rates and distributions of psychiatric disorders in the general population requires epidemiologic studies of samples of total populations within a geographically defined area. While there have been many such surveys[2] it is hazardous to use the existing data since the diagnostic criteria used have varied among studies and usually differ from the criteria used in genetic studies. Population surveys of mental illness conducted during the post-World War II period in the U.S. have attempted to deal with the unreliability of diagnosis not by making diagnostic distinctions but by instead using measures of overall impairment.[10,11] With the exception of one study recently completed but not yet published, U.S. studies using diagnostic categories were completed over 30 years ago. For more recent data, one must go to countries outside the United States, e.g., Scandinavia or Iceland, where, because of geographical and cultural differences, rates may not be at all comparable to those in the United States. The risk for manic-depressive illness estimated from these reviews is 1% to 2%.[12] Considering males and females separately, the estimated risks for major psychosis are 0.9% to 1.8% in males and 1.2% to 2.8% in females.[2] The lifetime risk for developing any affective illness (including "neurotic depression") is probably 6% to 10%.[13]

Application of the newer diagnostic methods in a recently completed study of a probability sample of a U.S. urban community showed a low frequency of bipolar affective disorder in the population but suggested that unipolar disorder may be much more common.[11] The estimation of population frequencies of mental disorders using the newer diagnostic methods will help considerably in interpreting future family studies.

THE EVIDENCE THAT GENES ARE INVOLVED

Twin Studies

Twin concordance rates for affective illness, based on six studies which met diagnostic and sampling standards, are 69.2% ± 4.8% for monozygotic (MZ) pairs and 13.3% ± 2.3% for dizygotic (DZ) pairs.[1] Assuming that intrapair environmental variances are the same for MZ and DZ twins, the higher concordance rate for affective illness in MZ twin pairs indicates a heritable disorder. Twelve pairs of MZ twins reared apart have been reported[14]; they show a concordance rate for affective illness that is comparable to that of MZ twins reared together—67% ± 14%. The presence of discordant MZ twin pairs, whether reared together or apart, can be considered evidence for the importance of nongenetic factors influencing the development of affective illness. This does not negate the suggestion, from the very high concordance rate of MZ twins and the considerably lower rate for DZ twins, that affective illness is a heritable disorder.

Twin studies have also been reviewed using the bipolar–unipolar classification of affective illness.[15] Pooling all studies gives the following pairwise concordance rates: for bipolar, 72% ± 5% for MZ and 14% ± 2% for DZ; for unipolar, 40% ± 13% for MZ and 11% ± 5% for DZ. The MZ concordances are significantly higher than those of the DZ for both disorders; the concordance for bipolar MZ twins is also significantly higher than that for unipolar MZ twins. In addition to suggesting that genetic factors are important, Allen[15] interprets the higher MZ concordance for bipolars as suggesting "genetic factors may be more important in the occurrence of bipolar illness than in unipolar illness." While we agree with the conclusion, those MZ concordances are not conclusive evidence. Concordance rates are not directly related to the magnitude of the genetic contribution.[16,17] To be interpretable genetically the concordances must be compared to the population incidences (as discussed above) in the context of a specific genetic model (to be discussed below). Thus, rigorous support for that interpretation requires that the sex- and diagnosis-specific general incidences for all of the populations in which the twin studies were done be compared to the sex- and diagnosis-specific concordances. Some consideration of various possible genetic models is also required.

Family Studies

The reported morbid risk of affective illness in first-degree relatives varies from study to study.[2,3] The variation is sufficiently large that it is unlikely to be due to random factors. Systematic differences in the studies (such as diagnostic and/or ascertainment criteria) or in the populations studied are more likely to be responsible.

Gershon et al.[1] have reviewed the literature for those family studies that consider unipolar and bipolar probands separately. The incidences of the two disorders among the first-degree relatives show some consistent patterns in most of the studies. Bipolar probands have both bipolar and unipolar relatives in roughly equal frequencies (about 7% and 8%, respectively). Unipolar probands have a low frequency of bipolar relatives (< 1%) and a lower incidence of unipolar relatives (6%) than do the bipolar probands. These data support the hypothesis that UP and BP affective disorders are also separable by the morbid risk of disease in relatives,[9,18] although there is considerable overlap since both types of probands can have both types of relatives.[19] More recently, Winokur[20] has proposed that UP is also heterogeneous and that two types can be defined based on type of illness in relatives. Others have proposed that bipolar disorder is heterogeneous and that those patients with full-blown manic episodes (Bipolar I) can be differentiated from those with milder hypomanic states (Bipolar II).

These morbidity risk data among first-degree relatives also indicate that the familial risk is probably higher than the population incidence. For bipolar illness a generally accepted figure for the morbidity risk of all affective disorder among first-degree relatives is about 15%. Even the highest population incidence estimate, 10%, is lower than most rates found in relatives of unipolar and bipolar depressives. The family-genetic study undertaken in Israel[21] was one of the few to collect both population data and data on a normal control group from the same population as their affected cases. In that study the lifetime incidence of affective disorder in the population was 2.4%, in the normal control group it was 0.77%, and in the relatives of both unipolar and bipolar probands it was 18%.

The bipolar–unipolar distinction is supported by twin studies, clinical observations, and pharmacological correlates. Both forms appear to be familial but may be due to different transmitted factors. The problems of overlap may be due to variable expression of the bipolar phenotype, which in the absence of mania would be confused with unipolar depression. Variable age of onset may magnify this problem. Other diagnostic subtypes may exist and be genetically distinct. There may be genetic heterogeneity within a clear diagnostic category.[20] But despite the methodologic variation among these and other studies and the strong suggestion of genetic heterogeneity, certain general conclusions seem possible: affective disorders run in families and can sometimes be traced through several generations.

WE ARE NOT SURE ABOUT MODES OF TRANSMISSION

Though the qualitative aspects of the data on the various affective disorders, as briefly summarized in the preceding paragraph, are strongly suggestive of genetic transmission, no single mode of inheritance has been unambiguously demonstrated for any subtype of the disorder.

X-LINKAGE

In the last few years it has been shown that, at least in some families, bipolar affective disorder seems to be transmitted from affected males primarily to daughters but from affected females to offspring of both sexes. This pattern not only adds evidence for genetic involvement but also suggests a specific mode of inheritance: X-linked dominant transmission; exceptions are attributed to slightly reduced penetrance in the heterozygous females. We do not find the evidence compelling that more than a small fraction, if any, of BP affective disorder is due to an X-linked locus.

The general incidences of both bipolar and unipolar affective illness appear to be higher in females than in males.[22] The male:female ratio in the population is about 1:1.6 for BP and 1:2.9 for UP.[1] One possible explanation for a greater frequency of a disorder in one sex is X-linkage, that is, the location of the relevant locus on the X chromosome. For an X-linked locus, if the trait is dominant, females (with two X chromosomes) are more commonly affected than males (with only one X chromosome). A rare X-linked dominant trait usually appears in the mother and all of the daughters of an affected male and in at least one parent and at least half of the children of an affected female. Incomplete penetrance—the occasional absence of the disease even though the necessary genes are present—would give rise to occasional exceptions and lower frequencies. The exact frequencies with which first-degree relatives are affected are also a function of the allele frequency in the population and of the mating pattern.

The results of family studies investigating X-linkage are conflicting. Perris[23] found a greater frequency of affected female relatives than affected male relatives for unipolar probands but not for bipolar probands. On the other hand, Helzer and Winokur[24] and Reich, Clayton, and Winokur[19] found data suggesting X-linkage for bipolar but not for unipolar depression: mothers of male BP probands were more often affected than the fathers. The inconsistency of studies has continued into recent work as well. Some studies[21,25] show no significant difference between female and male relatives of male probands; these studies suggest that the observed excess of affected mothers and daughters might simply be due to the generally present sex ratio in the affective illnesses.

The existence in all studies of some cases of apparent father-to-son transmission requires some modifications to a simple hypothesis of X-linkage. Two possibilities are (a) that not all cases are X-linked and (b) that by chance, or possibly because of assortative mating, the son actually inherited the predisposing gene from his mother.

Mendlewicz and Fleiss[26] have recently reviewed their studies of genetic linkage of known X-chromosome markers (protan with deutan color blindness, Xg blood group) and BP affective disorder and included informative pedigrees published by others. They report significant positive lods between both color-blindness loci and affective disorder for recombination rates of about 10%. The lod for Xg and affective disorder was positive at about 20% recombination and was at the borderline of significance. In these analyses unipolar relatives are assumed to differ from the proband only in diagnosis (as the result of random factors); the X-chromosome allele predisposing to affective disorder is assumed to be the same in the proband and in all affected relatives.

At first glance this seems to be compelling evidence for an X-linked locus. However, this X-linked locus apparently cannot account for all bipolar illness since, in the same study from which the pedigrees informative for linkage were selected, there were pedigrees with affected father–son pairs with no illness in the mother or her family.[27] Moreover, there are major reservations about accepting the lods and recombination rates actually calculated. For many of the pedigrees the maximum likelihood estimate for the recombination rate has not been correctly calculated.[28] Many families used in the original studies cannot be shown to be informative for linkage if more strict criteria are used. When those families are eliminated the lod score is not significant.

To date all published linkage studies of BP affective disorder have used published tables of lod scores.[29] In addition to containing one particular error,[30] those tables are inappropriate for use for several other reasons. The most obvious reason is the existence of incomplete penetrance; the recombination fraction estimated from the tables is actually a confounding of both recombination and incomplete penetrance. Another problem is that UP depression is generally considered in these analyses to be a manifestation of the BP genotype. Yet, we know that the UP form is much more frequent than BP and may reach 10% in a random population. Thus, it seems probable that some UP disorder will occur by chance among the relatives and be unrelated to linkage. Both of these problems in the analysis serve to make linkage harder to detect and suggest that the estimates of the recombination frequency are higher than the actual value.

This possible bias against linkage makes another aspect of the X-linkage studies even more disconcerting: the demonstration of close linkage to two different markers that are quite distant on the map. The resulting three-point linkage map is definitely not linear.[31] This inconsistency and the methodological problems in estimating recombination for this trait raise concerns over the reality of the apparent X-linkage. An additional complication of the X-linkage studies has also been mentioned[28]; in the reported linkage studies virtually all pedigrees have the reported bipolar allele in coupling with a color-blindness allele. A bias in this direction could be explained by a search only among affected males for color blindness; Gershon and Bunney[32] argue that this mechanism could not account for the entire discrepancy. This raises the possibility of linkage disequilibrium and/or an actual biochemical–physiological association between the two disorders.

The preceding and following criticisms notwithstanding, there are some large pedigrees which look very much like X-linked inheritance. When proper methods of pedigree analysis are applied to them, the question may be resolved. It seems likely that at least some bipolar illness is determined by an allele or alleles at an X-linked locus, but the proof is lacking.

Other Genetic Analyses

Another possible explanation of the different incidences in the two sexes is a differential interaction of genotype and environment depending on sex. A sex effect can be treated as a differential threshold with the less commonly affected sex having a higher threshold.[33,34] Those thresholds exist on a liability scale; the underlying liability is determined by a combination of both genetic and environmental factors. In this framework many of the commonly observed aspects of the sex effect can be explained by either of two types of inheritance: a polygenic model and a single-major-autosomal-locus model. The results of Uhlenhuth and Paykel[35] suggest that at the same level of stress females have more symptoms than males, an idea consistent with the concept of females' having a lower threshold and stress being a major component of liability.

The multiple-threshold approach, which uses either severity[35] or sex effect[33,34] to classify affected individuals, allows testing of some genetic hypotheses. Without the subdivision of affected into two groups, most sets of data on morbid risks to relatives cannot be used to discriminate between different genetic models.[16] Severity and a sex effect are logically similar as is seen by equating the less commonly affected sex to the more severe form of the disorder: both represent greater deviation from the mean. The underlying rationale of the two-threshold approach is that the rarer form is also more deviant genetically than the other. Consequently, a dominance variance may exist if there is a single major locus (SML) and may be different for the two types of the trait. A dominance variance is unlikely if the trait is polygenic, but, if any exists, the two types of the trait would give almost identical values because of the very slow decline in heterozygosity.[37]

Gershon et al.[38] have applied multiple-threshold models to unipolar (less severe form) and bipolar (more severe form) affective disorder data collected in Israel.[21] The models of Reich et al.[36] and Kidd et al.[33] were modified in this analysis to include a third threshold which defines milder related disturbances among relatives. The sex effect was not incorporated in the analysis since it was not pronounced in the Israeli data. The models were further modified to incorporate assortative mating and consanguinity. These modifications were felt necessary because of the documented occurrence of both in the population under study. The multifactorial (polygenic) model (MF) and the single-major-locus model (SML) both gave acceptable fits to the data.

Leckman and Gershon[39] have used the sex-effect versions of the MF and SML models to analyze data on families of bipolar probands. Because the analyses require that all relationship pairs also be specified by sex of both proband and relative, only four sets of data from the literature were suitable. Both the MF and SML models are autosomal models and make no allowance for X-linked inheritance. Thus, a true X-linked trait should be excluded by the analysis. Indeed, the data of Winokur and Clayton[40] and the data of Mendlewicz and Rainer[27] could not be explained by autosomal transmission with a sex effect. However, that same hypothesis could not be excluded for the data of Gershon et al.[21] and the data of Goetzl et al.[25] These results indirectly support the presence of X-linked transmission, or some other factor not included in or allowed by the assumptions of the models, in the data of Winokur and of

Mendlewicz. The analyses do not support X-linkage in the data of Goetzl and of Gershon.

Analyses by Van Eerdewegh, Gershon, and Van Eerdewegh[41] use an X-chromosome threshold model to analyze some of the same data sets. The data of Mendlewicz and Rainer[27] do not fit the model, but only a version which considered bipolar and unipolar identical disorders could be tested. The data of Winokur[40] and of Gershon[21] both gave the best fit to the version of the model which considered only bipolar relatives and classified unipolar relatives as unaffected.

Conclusion

All of the data and analyses discussed above emphasize the discrepancies among studies and the consequent uncertainty of genetic interpretations. Reasonably good evidence exists for a genetic component in bipolar disease. However, the mode(s) of transmission remain(s) unknown because of the likely presence of genetic, and possibly also diagnostic, heterogeneity. The evidence for genetic involvement in the unipolar disorders is less clear since there are fewer data. The data for other less severe forms of affective disorders are also less clear. A number of depressives fit neither the unipolar nor bipolar classification, e.g., schizoaffective depression, single-episode depression with no mania, so-called neurotic or mild depressions, and secondary depressives; for these, little or no data are available.

Unless a specific mode of genetic transmission can be demonstrated for a diagnostic group of affective disorders, the familial concentration that exists could be attributed to cultural transmission or environmental correlations among relatives. These are both alternatives to genetic transmission that cannot be ignored.

THE DATA WE NEED

In the absence of information on a biochemical aberration, how can other types of studies be designed so that they yield reliable, less ambiguous data? Such studies must meet the following minimum requirements.

1. Diagnostically homogeneous subgroups need to be considered separately whenever possible. Though this does not eliminate the possibility of genetic heterogeneity, it is a major step toward minimizing it.

2. The relatives need to be very accurately diagnosed and classified, irrespective of the diagnosis of the proband.

3. The diagnostic criteria used must be standardized and their reliability and validity must have been demonstrated.

4. The same diagnostic criteria used for probands must also be uniformly applied to relatives and a representative population sample. Only in this way can the risks in relatives be compared to the morbid risk of the psychiatric disorders in the general population.

5. The general population and the probands should derive from relatively the same culture and be studied at the same time, so as to minimize cultural and temporal variation.

6. Diagnostic classification of relatives should be based on direct interview. Whenever interviewing is not possible, multiple informants should be used to verify the data obtained.

7. Interviewing and diagnosis of the relatives must be done by investigators who are blind to the status of the proband.

8. Large samples are required to discriminate among genetic models. Certainly many families must be studied. However, if there exists genetic heterogeneity, it is probably necessary to use pedigree analysis on individual large families, ideally multigenerational families with large sibships.

9. The existence of assortative mating and consanguinity must be considered. If either exists, it must be considered in the analyses.

The above criteria are also important for studies of biochemical factors that may be relevant. The ultimately important problem is defining the types of genetic (biochemical) susceptibility and the specific nongenetic "stresses" that interact with each. This information can only be obtained from both biochemical and diagnostic data on biologically related individuals. Even if the genetics is simple, e.g., just one locus, heterogeneity for susceptibility can exist and complex genotype–environment interactions are expected.[42]

One other powerful research strategy is the search for genetic linkage. Unambiguous demonstration of close linkage between a marker locus and a locus for high susceptibility to illness provides proof of genetic involvement and represents significant progress in resolving gene–environment interactions. Linkage studies should not be confined to bipolars and X-linked markers. Families with unipolar disorder, both severe and mild, and familes with BP, both with and without affected father–son pairs, should be studied for linkage to all possible marker loci.

Studies currently under way in several centers in the United States incorporate almost all of these features, including biochemical studies in families and genetic linkage studies. However, it may be another three or four years before the data will be collected and preliminary analyses completed. One hopes that at that time we shall be closer to understanding the genetics of affective disorders.

ACKNOWLEDGMENTS

This work was supported in part by grant MH 28274-01 from the Center for Epidemiologic Studies of the National Institute of Mental Health. The authors wish to thank Judith R. Kidd for her editorial assistance.

REFERENCES

1. Gershon ES, Bunney, WE Jr, Leckman JF, Van Eerdewegh M, DeBauche BA: The inheritance of affective disorders: A review of data and hypotheses. *Behav. Genet.* *6:*227–261, 1976.
2. Perris C: Frequency and hereditary aspects of depression. In: Gallant DM, Simpson GM (eds) *Depression: Behavioral, Biochemical, Diagnostic and Treatment Concepts,* pp. 75–107. New York, Spectrum, 1976.
3. Tsuang MT: Genetics of affective disorder. In: Mendels J (ed) *Psychobiology of Depression,* pp. 85–100. New York, John Wiley and Sons, 1976.
4. Gershon ES, Targum SD, Kessler LR, Mazure CM, Bunney WE: Genetic studies and biologic strategies in the affective disorders. In: *Prog. Med. Genet.* (in press).
5. Spitzer RL, Endicott J, Robins E: Clinical criteria for psychiatric diagnosis and the DSM-III. *Am. J. Psychiatry 132:*1187–1192, 1975.
6. Kramer M: Cross national study of diagnosis of the mental disorders: Origin of the problem. *Am. J. Psychiatry 125*(suppl.):1–11, 1969.
7. Zubin J: Cross national study of diagnosis of the mental disorders: Methodology and planning. *Am. J. Psychiatry 125*(suppl.):12–20, 1969.
8. Robins E, Guze S: Establishment of diagnostic validity in psychiatric illness: Its application to schizophrenia. *Am. J. Psychiatry 127:*107–111, 1970.
9. Leonhard K: *Aufteilung der Endogenen Psychosen* (1st ed.). Berlin, 1957.
10. Weissman MM, Klerman GL: Epidemiology of mental disorders: Emerging trends. Submitted for publication.
11. Weissman MM, Meyers JK: The New Haven Survey 1967–75: Depressive symptoms and diagnosis. To be published in the Proceedings of the Conference of The Society for Life History Research in Psychopathology, Fort Worth, Texas, 1976.
12. Klerman GL, Barrett J: The affective disorders: Clinical and epidemiological aspects. In: Gershon S, Shopsin B (eds) *Lithium: Its Role in Psychiatric Research and Treatment.* New York, Plenum Press, 1973.
13. Silverman C: *The Epidemiology of Depression.* Johns Hopkins University Press, Baltimore, 1968.

14. Price J: The genetics of depressive behavior. In: Coppen A, Walk A (eds) *Recent Developments in Affective Disorders. Br. J. Psychiatry* Special Publication No. 2, pp. 37–54, 1968.
15. Allen MG: Twin studies of affective illness. *Arch. Gen. Psychiatry 33:*1476–1478, 1976.
16. Matthysse SW, Kidd KK: Estimating the genetic contribution to schizophrenia. *Am. J. Psychiatry 133:*185–191, 1976.
17. Smith C: Concordance in twins: Methods and interpretation. *Am. J. Hum. Genet. 26:* 454–466, 1974.
18. Leonhard K, Korff I, Schulz H: Die Temperamente in den Familien der monopolaren und bipolaren phasischen Psychosen. *Psychiat. Neurol. 143:*416–434, 1962.
19. Reich T, Clayton PJ, Winokur G: Family history studies: V. The genetics of mania. *Am. J. Psychiatry 125:*1358–1370, 1969.
20. Winokur G: Depression spectrum disease: Description and family study. *Compr. Psychiatry 13:*3–8, 1972.
21. Gershon ES, Mark A, Cohen N, Belizon N, Baron M, Knobe KE: Transmitted factors in the morbid risk of affective disorders: A controlled study. *J. Psychiat. Res. 12:*283–299, 1975.
22. Weissman MM, Klerman GL: Sex differences and the epidemiology of depression. *Arch. Gen. Psychiatry 34:*98–111, 1977.
23. Perris C: Abnormality on paternal and maternal sides: Observations in bipolar (manic-depressive) and unipolar depressive psychoses. *Br. J. Psychiatry 118:*207–210, 1971.
24. Helzer J, Winokur, G: A family interview study of male manic-depressives. *Arch. Gen. Psychiatry 31:*73–77, 1974.
25. Goetzl U, Green R, Whybrow P, Jackson R: X-linkage revisited—A further family history study of manic-depressive illness. *Arch. Gen. Psychiatry 31:*665–672, 1974.
26. Mendlewicz J, Fleiss JL: Linkage studies with X-chromosome markers in bipolar (manic-depressive) and unipolar (depressive) illnesses. *Biol. Psychiatry 9:*261–294, 1974.
27. Mendlewicz J, Rainer JD: Morbidity risk and genetic transmission in manic-depressive illness. *Am. J. Hum. Genet. 26:*692–701, 1974.
28. Gershon ES, Bunney WE: The question of X-linkage in bipolar manic-depressive illness. *J. Psychiat. Res. 13:*99–117, 1977.
29. Edwards JH: The analysis of X-linkage. *Ann. Hum. Genet. 34:*229–250, 1971.
30. Gershon ES, Matthysse SW: X-linkage: Ascertainment through doubly ill probands. *J. Psychiat. Res.,* 1977 (in press).
31. Matthysse SW: In: Review of pedigrees informative for linkage to Xg. *Neurosci. Res. Prog. Bull. 14:*51, 1976.
32. Gershon ES, Bunney WE: Association between manic-depressive illness and color blindness. *Neurosci. Res. Program Bull. 14:*49–50, 1976.
33. Kidd KK, Reich T, Kessler S: A genetic analysis of stuttering suggesting a single major locus. *Genetics 74:*S 137 (abstract), 1973.
34. Kidd KK, Spence MA: Genetic analyses of pyloric stenosis suggesting a specific maternal effect. *J. Med. Genet. 13:*290–294, 1976.
35. Uhlenhuth EH, Paykel ES: Symptom intensity and life events. *Arch. Gen. Psychiatry 28:*473–477, 1973.
36. Reich T, James JW, Morris CA: The use of multiple thresholds in determining the mode of transmission of semi-continuous traits. *Ann. Hum. Genet. (London) 36:*163–184, 1972.
37. Cavalli–Sforza LL, Kidd KK: Genetic models for schizophrenia. *Neurosci. Res. Program Bull. 10:*406–419, 1972.

38. Gershon ES, Baron M, Leckman J: Genetic models of the transmission of affective disorders. *J. Psychiat. Res. 12*:301–317, 1975.
39. Leckman JF, Gershon ES: Autosomal models of sex effect in bipolar-related major affective illness. *J. Psychiat. Res. 13*(4), 1977.
40. Winokur G, Clayton P: Family history studies. I. Two types of affective disorders separated according to genetic and clinical factors. In: Wortis IJ (ed) *Recent Advances in Biological Psychiatry*, Vol. 9, pp. 35–50. New York, Plenum Press, 1967.
41. Van Eerdewegh M, Gershon ES, Van Eerdewegh P: X-chromosome models of bipolar illness. *Sci. Proc. Am. Psychiat. Assoc. 129* (summary):124–125, 1976.
42. Matthysse SW, Kidd KK: Genetic principles in defining homogeneous subgroups of the schizophrenias. In: Akiskal H (ed) *Toward a Biological Classification of Psychiatric Disorders*. New York, Spectrum, 1977.

6

Drug Therapy of Depression

NATHAN S. KLINE

The classification of depressive disorders is far from settled. The categories I present differ from those of others because, at present, agreement does not exist as to how depressive disorders should be classified. I hope that the next few years will provide clear, final, and definitive biochemical indices to the biological classification of depression. Such a classification would enable us finally and clearly to separate the subtypes of depression and to prescribe specific therapies for each. Some 2000 years ago, Leucippus authored a very pertinent statement. He said, "Where there is ignorance, theories abound." One hopes that this volume will help reduce the number of such theories.

There are still, however, many contradictory points of view. A friend of mine came to a conference in which I was participating; at the beginning I asked him why he had come and he said because he was confused. At the end of the conference I asked him if his confusion had been straightened out. He said "No, I'm still confused, but it's a higher order of confusion." Part of our own confusion arises from the fact that everyone experiences some depression at one time or another. Some of this depression may be a normal reaction to external stress (existential depression) and some of it may in fact be a form of depressive illness. Since everyone experiences depression, it makes all psychiatrists *and* all laymen experts on depression.

There are moods and fashions in depression and at times it is fashionable to be depressed and at other times it is not. In the seventeenth century there was a period during the Reformation when depression was out, whereas in the Elizabethan period depression was in. It was during this period that the expression "the happy moron" originated, with the idea that anyone who is happy must be moronic and anyone

NATHAN S. KLINE • Rockland Research Institute, Orangeburg, New York.

who is sensitive or intelligent would necessarily be melancholic. In fact, toward the end of the nineteenth century Goethe published a book called *Werther's Leiden* or *The Sorrows of Werther*, in which the protagonist was in love with a married woman and, quite in contrast to today's society, he didn't even mention to her how he felt. Because he believed his case was hopeless, he committed suicide. The publication of this widely read book literally caused an epidemic of suicides throughout a good portion of Europe.

A question frequently asked is, "Is depression more frequent today than it was ten or twenty years ago?" Statistics on treated cases would certainly seem to indicate that to be true in the United States. I know from personal correspondence with Professor Snezhnevsky at the Institute of Psychiatry in Moscow that the number of cases in the USSR diagnosed as depression has also increased markedly. However, there are grounds for believing that the incidence of depression itself may not have increased but merely the awareness and hence the diagnosis. There is the additional factor that, if treatment for a condition is available, it makes sense to make the diagnosis, whereas if no treatment is available, then one tends to neglect the diagnosis. I think the availability of treatment has a good deal to do with the recent increase in depressive diagnoses. A related point is that, in the less developed countries the incidence of depression appears to be pretty much the same as it is in the Western world. On balance, as far as I can tell from my consultant work in Africa and Southeast Asia, there has not been any real increase in the incidence but merely in the use of the depressive diagnoses.

Culture does, to some degree, modify the way depression is perceived and presented. In Indonesia where we computerized the record-keeping of all the twenty-three public hospitals, we found the incidence of depression to be about the same as in the United States. However, interestingly, in a five-year review of the Indonesian hospital data we computed, there is no case of a native Indonesian having either attempted or committed suicide. The Dutch, who were located there, were committing suicide at about the same rate as they were in Amsterdam or Rotterdam, and the Japanese who had returned after the war were committing suicide even more enthusiastically than they were in Tokyo and Yokohama. Obviously, there are culturally determined modes of expression of depressive illness. In Africa, for instance, depression tends to show itself primarily in somatic symptoms rather than in the expressions of guilt and remorse which are fairly common in

Western society. I think this has a good deal to do with the general structure of the society and the general mores. In the Western world we take the attitude of *mea culpa,* "I am to blame"—also, *mea lauda,* "I am to be praised." In other words, what happens to us is largely an individual matter and if things do go wrong we have feelings of depression and we tend to attach feelings of guilt to them. In societies such as those in West Africa and Southeast Asia the primary identification is a group one, so that an individual thinks of himself or herself first as a member of a group and only later, if at all, as an individual.

The group social structure and the belief in magic, which is strong in these cultures, both combine to remove from the individual the feelings of helplessness and hopelessness so characteristic of depression in Western cultures. The individual is never totally isolated and alone in the first place, while a belief in magic carries with it the possibility of instant solutions to even highly unpleasant situations.

Despite these cultural differences in the manifestations and symptoms, the types of depression, as I see them, occur in all cultures. The first of these, as already mentioned, is existential depression. This is the type of depression which we all experience. Many patients with more severe depressions are able, they tell me, to distinguish between what I mean by existential depression and the type of depression which calls for psychiatric treatment. Existential depression is the type which results from either the Democrats or the Republicans getting elected, from the right or the wrong baseball team winning the ball game, or from unpleasant or traumatic events in one's personal life. It covers a wide spectrum of mildly severe depressive responses to outside events.

The second group of depressions are those which are designated as "secondary depressions." These are depressions which result from some clearly identifiable cause. Such depressions are usually not studied by investigators such as Dr. Schildkraut because their known biological or chemical causes would confound such data. A good example of the secondary depression is the depression secondary to the use of reserpine or Rauwolfia compounds; these produce depression in about 15% of individuals being treated for hypertension. The use of steroids and oral contraceptives also is associated with the onset of depression in some individuals. Antibiotic drugs such as the sulfonamides, methenamine mandelate, and other drugs will occasionally produce depression. It is important to recognize the relationship between drug therapies and such secondary depressions while taking medical histories from psychiatric patients, since the simple withdrawal of the offending medication is often sufficient to relieve the patient of the symptoms, and the need for psychopharmacological intervention disappears.

Almost any viral disorder will bring about a depression in a fair number of individuals. Anyone who has had infectious mononucleosis is aware of how much depression this illness can induce. I managed to have my infectious mononucleosis during my last year in medical school. I already had an experimental bent at that time and I asked the internist caring for me to save a pint or two of blood to see if, after I recovered, I would feel as lousy again when he retransfused me with it. Unfortunately, he was not an experimentalist so there is a piece of research which still remains to be done. But depression does appear, in most viral disorders, to be a sequela.

Lots of operative procedures can also produce depression. Since my own analyst was Paul Schilder, I obviously would attribute this to distortion of the body image. Whether such depressions are totally psychological or whether, as the Russians would argue, there is a biological, physiological, or pharmacological factor involved in anesthesia or trauma which may produce the depression, it is important to know that depression often follows operations. Treatment again should be deferred until one is sure there will not be a fairly rapid spontaneous remission.

One should also not forget that there are physical disorders such as anemia, avitaminosis, and a whole variety of other physical conditions which also produce depression, e.g., Wilson's disease. Hence a physical evaluation of depressed individuals is important.

There are obviously some situations in which the depression appears secondary to major life events, but it is difficult to tell whether the stresses inolved are dynamic or biological. Postpartum depressions associated with childbirth are such an example. I would ordinarily attribute these to the biological changes associated with childbirth, were it not for the fact that I have found similar depressions in authors who have given birth to a book. Two authors of successful first novels, Ross Lockridge, the author of *Raintree County,* and Thomas Heggen, the author of *Mr. Roberts,* both committed suicide following successful publication of their works. I have now had a fair number of authors as patients and find that they not infrequently have depressions following completion of such works. The individual feels that he is "produced out" and that he will never be able to work again. The psychological solution to this problem is to get the author so involved in his next piece of work that, when the earlier book is published, he is all wrapped up in opus number two. This might also work for ordinary pregnancies, but I can't find an obstetrician to cooperate in the research.

Secondary depressions also occur in a setting of other diagnosable *psychiatric* illnesses. Perhaps the most common of these is the depression young people often develop when they become aware of symptoms of schizophrenia within themselves. This depression often seems reactive to their disturbed inner state rather than part of the schizophrenia itself. Patients with obsessive compulsive disorders, recurrent anxiety attacks, or marked organic brain damage not infrequently also develop a secondary depression.

The other side of this coin is perhaps even more important. This is the fact that there are two conditions which are frequently misdiagnosed but which really do constitute depression. If these are missed, it is of therapeutic significance. One of these is the failure to distinguish between depression and schizophrenia. The occurrence of auditory hallucinations and delusions is relatively common in very severe depressions. Many cases with such symptoms are automatically classified as schizophrenia and are then treated with phenothiazines or related major tranquilizers; if anything, such drugs retard the patient's recovery and may prevent spontaneous remissions. To avoid this mistake, clinicians should look for other stigmata of schizophrenia (e.g., cognitive defects) before making the diagnosis. One should not make the automatic assumption that hallucinations and delusions mean schizophrenia.

The other situation in which depression is missed is much more important since it occurs even more frequently, that is, in an individual with borderline arteriosclerosis or senility. When such an individual does become depressed, the high probability is that what one will see symptomatically is not the depression but the organic symptoms (pseudodementia). The occurrence of the depression interferes with the compensatory process which normally exists in aging individuals to cope with mild to moderate organic defects. As we grow older, we forget names and places and facts and figures. We usually can figure some way around these, but if one is depressed, the compensatory process is weak or absent. The individuals, hence, are very frequently diagnosed as arteriosclerotic and senile and, since we have no adequate treatment for such brain defects, they are let to go pretty much untreated. One should always look for the presence of depression in any arteriosclerotic or senile individual and, in many cases, even though there is not a clear-cut occurrence of depression, it is worth treating the patient as though he or she were depressed since a surprising number of such patients do recoup. Often six to eight weeks are required before there is evidence of real improvement on antidepressant drugs in elderly patients; thus one should persist with such therapy longer than one might in younger patients.

A proportion of the depressions seen in general clinical practice occur in individuals who also have had manic attacks. Such depressions are usually called "bipolar" and are identical with the older diagnosis of manic-depressive illness. However, the vast majority of the depressions seen in office practice and in hospitals are, to my way of thinking, unipolar. Much has been written about the differences between neurotic and psychotic depressions and between reactive and endogenous depressions. On the basis of experience, I tend to see unipolar depression as a single entity which varies in severity and manifestations for a variety of reasons, one of which is the personality of the individual in whom the depression occurs.

Obviously, neurotic individuals who develop depression will complicate their depression because of their neurotic features. As will be noted below, I tend to handle such patients differently in therapy.

The above rather simple classification of depressions into (1) existential, (2) secondary, (3) bipolar, (4) unipolar, and (5) neurotic is adequate for most therapeutic purposes. When I evaluate a patient with depressive symptoms, there are a number of questions I routinely ask, and the first of these is, "Is medication needed at all?" Existential depressions, which are manifestations of normal mourning or normal grief or normal responses to environmental stress, should ordinarily not be treated pharmacologically. Similarly, if the depression appears secondary to a virus infection or to the ingestion of reserpine, either no treatment is indicated or there should be withdrawal of the medication. At some point, if depressive symptoms persist or become more severe, specific therapy may be indicated, but initially, in depressions which present as either existential or secondary depressions, no antidepressant therapy may be needed.

The question exists, "Is electroconvulsive therapy the treatment of choice?" I admit to being prejudiced about ECT for a variety of reasons, one of which is that most of the medications which I administer I try myself. I must admit I have not tried ECT to see what the effect is like, nor have I tried lobotomy. I suspect that the prejudice which I have against ECT is fairly common among patients; if patients dislike a therapy of their illness, they may try to deny the illness when it recurs and not return for necessary treatment early enough. For this reason, I prefer the use of medication to the use of ECT. Nevertheless, there are two clear-cut indications for the use of ECT. One of these is in the acutely suicidal patient. Despite the views of Dr. Szasz and Dr. Laing and others about the civil rights of patients, it is my feeling that the unrestricted right to commit suicide is something one must question. An actually suicidal patient, who in your opinion is clearly suffering from an illness, may require ECT since the drugs take about three weeks to begin to produce real improvement. Also, there is a danger period of increased suicidal risk as the patient begins to improve. This suicidal danger is a clear-cut indication for the use of ECT.

ECT is also indicated in a small number of patients who show minimal or no improvement on more conventional drug therapies and for whom the addition of a small number of shock treatments makes a substantial difference. I have one patient now who does well on medication but at the end of four or five weeks begins to show increasing depression; at this point, one or two ECTs will bring him back to a socially functioning level. ECT without medication has no effect.

Thus, I believe there are indications for ECT but I do not believe that it is the sole or major treatment to be used in depressed patients. Although it may be more rapid acting than drug therapies in acute situations, patients not infrequently relapse shortly after ECT is stopped and the response to repeated courses of treatment tends to become less consistent and predictable over time.

Having decided that drugs are indicated, one must look at the contraindications rather than the indications for particular drug therapies. Against the use of the tricyclic antidepressants is the presence or history of thrombophlebitis or of increased intraocular pressure including narrow-angle glaucoma. The tricyclics may also aggravate hyperthyroidism, and the presence of a recent myocardial infarct also makes the use of tricyclic antidepressants unwise. Against the use of a monamine oxidase inhibitor is the presence of a pheochromocytoma, a history of a chronic liver disorder, a consistent trend toward alcoholism (because the combination of MAOIs and alcohol is not a good one) and, on occasion, marked hypotension. Minimal hypotension is not a contraindication. Another important consideration is the presence of organic cerebral disorder of any kind because such individuals tend to be very sensitive to all medications. Drugs can be used but they should be used cautiously, beginning with small dosages. The other question is whether the patient has responded to prior treatment with one or another of the drugs. There is strong evidence that individuals in the same family tend to respond to the same medication. In the *Journal of the American Medical Association* a few years ago, I reported on a set of identical twins neither of whom knew what the other was receiving, one being treated by myself and one by one of the associates in my office; it turned out that they specifically responded only to a single MAO inhibitor. Obviously, if a patient has responded well to a particular medication, it is a good one with which to begin treatment a second time. I should also point out, however, that in some cases the individual may respond to a drug one time and not another, so that failure to respond does not mean that the individual has become drug resistant. It merely means that he is resistant to that particular medication on that particular occasion.

Our own method of proceeding is to start with one of the tricyclic antidepressants. The decision as to which tricyclic antidepressant to use is determined in large part by the degree of sedation which is required. The antidepressants range from those that have a stimulant effect such as protriptyline (Vivactil), which has side effects resembling the amphetamines, to the more sedative drugs on the other extreme: medications such as amitriptyline (Elavil), nortriptyline (Aventyl), and doxepin (Sinequan or Adepin). In the center, which is the region where most treatment occurs, are imipramine (Tofranil) and desipramine (Pertofrane or Norpramin). These are generally effective in a majority of cases.

I avoid the sedative antidepressant drugs in clinical situations where sedation would obviously constitute a hazard. One example of this sort is the airline pilot who has depression which requires treatment but who is operating complex machinery in a high-risk situation. In such a patient I would use a stimulant drug such as protriptyline. I would tend to use nonsedative drugs also in situations where supervision of the patient is not available. For example, if a grandmother lives all by herself, medication which makes her sleepy may cause her to drop off to sleep with a cigarette burning—an unhealthy situation.

Since it is sometimes difficult to predict which drug will cause sedation in any individual patient, in patients in whom sedation would be a real risk I tend to initiate treatment with a low dose and to observe the patient's reaction, before pushing the dose upward.

A similar approach is called for in patients who, for personality reasons, seem unlikely to tolerate the side effects which are commonly experienced when antidepressant drugs are administered. As noted above, I believe that neurotic individuals can experience depressive episodes. When both conditions are present, then both diagnoses should be made since such individuals tend to be hypersensitive or at least hyperreactive to side effects. They will complain that the dryness of the mouth is intolerable, become preoccupied with constipation secondary to drug administration, or experience a wide range of other symptoms—dizziness, drowsiness, headaches, etc.—and will then complain bitterly about them, weaving the side effects into the depressive illness. Although such individuals can be managed with reassurance and support, if a depressed patient is identified as clearly neurotic, it is wise to use a medication that is low in side effects, to introduce it at a much lower dose than one would ordinarily use, and to raise it gradually to avoid the patient's overreaction to side effects. In such patients it may be possible to arrive at a therapeutic dose without having the patient rebel against the side effects and discontinue treatment. For the majority of patients, the choice of a specific antidepressant medication may not be the major problem. In the practice we conduct in mid-Manhattan, we have been seeing about 700 patients a year, of whom almost 80% were depressed. Most of these had already been treated by someone else and 20% were referred to us by other psychiatrists or psychologists or family doctors. The major errors made were not in the selection of the drug. The major errors made were twofold: (1) the dosage tended to be too low, the referring physician having tried too hard to avoid side effects. In terms of imipramine dosage, the usual dosage range in depressed patients referred to us was somewhere between 30 and 75 mg a day. We find that 150 mg a day is the average dose necessary to relieve depression and we have no hesitancy in going to much higher doses—up to 225 to 300 mg a day when necessary. (2) The other major mistake is to expect the depression to improve too soon. It does take 3 weeks for improvement to begin in most cases. We try to emphasize this to our patients so there is no misunderstanding on this issue. Normally we would continue treatment with the first drug for a month. If there were no signs of improvement at that time, we would try a second tricyclic. If this drug also failed to help the patient, we would next try one of the monoamine oxidase inhibitors. Although available treatments—the tricyclics or the MAO inhibitors—are a substantial help in the majority of depressed patients, the drugs suffer from a distressing slowness in onset of action and from a variety of side effects, contraindications, and other difficulties. It is therefore reassuring to know that new developments continue to occur which may have relevance to the future treatment of depression in this country. Some compounds are now in general use overseas. Tryptophan, a probable precursor of serotonin in the brain, is in general use in England and has been used successfully by our group in New York in over 500 patients. Ludiomil (maprotiline), a tetracyclic antidepressant, may also be a specific norepinephrine reuptake blocker and may therefore be uniquely valuable in depressions related to norepinephrine deficiency in the brain. It is in general use in Europe and in clinical trial in this country. Trazodone, another nontricyclic antidepressant, is on the market in Italy and is in early clinical trial in this country. Again, it may be a bit more effective and a good bit faster acting than available drugs on the market in the United States.

There has been recent interest in the use of sleep deprivation as a way of improving the symptoms of depression. A recent study has even suggested that sleep deprivation on the first day of drug therapy speeds response to the drug. Studies of thyroid-releasing hormone (TRH) suggest this polypeptide found in the central nervous system may have a stimulant or antidepressant effect in man under some circumstances, suggesting the possibility that this or other polypeptides may have a future role in the treatment of depression. In addition, more biochemical research of the type carried out by Dr. Schildkraut and Dr. Goodwin may well lead us to more specific, rational therapies for depression based on identified biochemical defects or excesses specific in depressed patients.

7

Further Notes on Drug Therapy

JONATHAN O. COLE

I agree with most of Dr. Kline's statements about the drug treatment of depression. For the benefit of the clinicians reading this section, I am providing a table (Table I) of the antidepressants available on a prescription basis in the United States at this time and their approximate effective dosages, as well as the dosage forms in which each is available. The reader who is also a careful student of package inserts will note that some of my dosage ranges slightly exceed the upper dosage recommended by the FDA and the company. Higher dosages should only be tried in patients who failed to respond at lower levels and showed no undesirable side effects at those dosages. In older patients who have had prior cardiovascular disease, consultation with an internist should be held and an electrocardiogram should be obtained before exceeding the upper "recommended" dosage. Where feasible, drug blood levels or platelet monoamine oxidase activity levels should be checked (see below).

In selecting a tricyclic drug and a dose of that drug, I have the same concerns as does Dr. Kline. In working with patients or active students (e.g., in law school), I try to avoid oversedating the patient. I often do this by starting the drug at a very low dose, if it is sedating (e.g., amitriptyline, 25 mg, h.s.) and if the patient also has insomnia, or I begin with 10 mg of protriptyline, if the patient has had bad experiences with sedation after taking other antidepressants.

I find that some outpatients, both old and young, get a good drug response on dosages as low as 50 mg of imipramine. In a referral practice, it is more usual to see other physicians' drug failures; as Kline says, many of these need simply a higher dose of the same drug and respond to a dosage between 150 and 300 mg a day. Within the tricyclics, I demonstrate my belief in the Schildkraut biochemical data by prescrib-

JONATHAN O. COLE • McLean Hospital, Belmont, Massachusetts.

TABLE I. PERTINENT DATA ON ANTIDEPRESSANT DRUGS[a]

Generic name	Trade name	Preparations available
Tricyclic antidepressants		
1. Imipramine hydrochloride	Tofranil Presamine SK-Pramine Imavate	Tablets: 10 mg, 25 mg, 50 mg Injection (I.M.): 12.5 mg/cc
2. Imipramine pamoate	Tofranil-PM	Capsules: 75 mg, 100 mg, 125 mg, 150 mg
3. Desipramine	Norpramin Pertofrane	Tablets or capsules: 25 mg, 50 mg
4. Amitriptyline	Elavil Endep	Tablets: 10 mg, 25 mg, 50 mg, 75 mg, 100 mg, 150 mg Injection (I.M.): 10 mg/cc
5. Nortriptyline	Aventyl	Capsules: 10 mg, 25 mg Liquid: 10 mg/5cc
6. Protriptyline	Vivactyl	Tablets: 5 mg, 10 mg
7. Doxepin	Sinequan	Capsules: 10 mg, 25 mg, 50 mg, 100 mg Concentrate: 10 mg/cc
Monoamine oxidase inhibitors		
1. Isocarboxazid	Marplan	Tablets: 10 mg
2. Phenelzine	Nardil	Tablets: 15 mg
3. Tranylcypromine	Parnate	Tablets: 10 mg
Stimulants		
1. Amphetamine	Benzedrine	Tablets: 5 mg, 10 mg Sustained-action capsules: 15 mg
2. Dextroamphetamine	Dexedrine	Tablets: 5 mg Sustained-action capsules: 5 mg, 10 mg, 15 mg Elixir: 5 mg/5 cc
3. Deanol	Deaner	Tablets: 25 mg, 100 mg
4. Methamphetamine	Desoxyn	Tablets: 2.5 mg, 5 mg Sustained-action tablets: 5 mg, 10 mg, 15 mg
5. Methylphenidate	Ritalin	Tablets: 5 mg, 10 mg, 20 mg

[a]We are grateful to Barbara Ameer for her preparation of this table.

ing imipramine, a "noradrenergic" tricyclic, for depression in bipolar patients and amitriptyline (a "serotonergic" tricyclic) in chronic characterological depressions, unless there is a good reason to do otherwise.

If a patient fails on any of the other tricyclics, which are all rather noradrenergic, I try amitriptyline, and, if a patient fails on amitriptyline,

I will next try imipramine or perhaps doxepin, if insomnia is a real problem, or protriptyline, if sedation–retardation is a major difficulty.

If the patient cannot tolerate a tricyclic because of peripheral anticholinergic effects—dry mouth, blurred vision, difficulty urinating, or constipation—urecholine, 25 mg, or occasionally 50 mg, t.i.d., may be added as a peripheral cholinergic drug.[1]

Alternately, based on Snyder's report on the relative anticholinergic potencies of tricyclics,[2] one can shift the patient to desipramine as the least anticholinergic (*in vitro*) of these drugs. Or, of course, one can continue therapy at a lower dose of the same drug.

For central anticholinergic side effects—thought blocking, memory problems, slight confusion, or disorientation—one must lower the dose of the drug; I tend to stop the drug for 24 hours or until the symptoms clear.[3] For the adventurous physician, 1 mg of physostigmine parenterally will reverse the central anticholinergic effects rapidly, though transiently (for 1 or 2 hours).[4]

In older patients, I start at even lower dosages (e.g., 10 mg of imipramine) and raise the dose more gingerly. For patients over 60, a pretreatment EKG is wise to have. For patients with heart disease, internal medical consultation–collaboration is desirable and perhaps the EKG should be monitored. In the absence of better alternatives and in the presence of a little reassuring data, I tend to start with doxepin in cardiac patients.[5]

I hope and believe that the t-wave changes often seen in EKGs after tricyclics are benign, but the bundle-branch block or prolongations of the QRS interval are more worrisome; there is no convincing epidermiological data demonstrating that any tricyclic in ordinary dosages causes morbidity (real medical complications) at a higher rate than would occur without tricyclic drug administration.

If patients fail to improve to 150 to 200 mg of the higher dose tricyclics for 2 to 3 weeks and have no or minimal side effects, I go higher. If at 300 mg for one week the same situation remains, I would work up toward 400 mg.

I hope that tricyclic blood levels soon become generally available. Data to date suggest that levels less than 150 ng (nanograms) may be inadequate. For nortriptyline, but not for the others, there is a suggestion of a therapeutic window (patients with blood levels over 150 ng and under 40 ng both do worse than patients in the 40 to 150 range).[6,7]

In patients who don't respond to tricyclics and have clear endogenous features, electroconvulsive therapy is the logical next step. Between four and twelve treatments are necessary. Unilateral electrode placement and use of barbiturate anesthesia and muscle relaxants avoid almost all the risks and discomforts of this therapy.[8] It may well be the logical first step for clearly paranoid depressions.[9] If such patients won't consent to ECT, treating paranoia first with an antipsychotic and then adding a tricyclic later, after the paranoid agitation has decreased, is a reasonable alternative.

If the depressed patient is nonendogenous, a trial on an MAOI is indicated, as Kline suggests. The monitoring of platelet MAO levels to titrate dose against percent inhibition should be helpful in adjusting dosage. I would warn, however, against attempts to achieve very rapid MAO inhibition by running the dose up rapidly (e.g., to 60 mg phenelzine q.d. in 3 days). My early attempts to speed the antidepressant effects of MAOIs led only to severe and persistent, agitated insomnia.

REFERENCES

1. Everett HC: The use of bethanecholchloride with tricyclic antidepressants. *Am. J. Psychiatry 132:*1202–1204, 1975.
2. Snyder SH, Yamamura HI: Antidepressants and the nuscarinic acetylcholine receptor. *Arch. Gen. Psychiatry 34:*236–239, 1977.
3. Cole JO, Schatzberg A: Memory difficulty and tricyclic antidepressants. *McLean Hosp. J. 1:*102–107, 1976.
4. Granacher RP, Baldaressarini RJ: Physostigmine. *Arch. Gen. Psychiatry 32:*375–380, 1975.
5. Goldberg HL, Finnerty RJ, Cole JO: The effect of doxepin in the aged: An interim report on memory changes and electrocardiographic findings. In: Mendels J (ed) *Sinequan (Doxepin Hydrochloride): A Monograph of Recent Clinical Studies.* Excerptá Medica, 1975.
6. Glassman AH, Perel JM, Shostak M, Kantor SJ, Fleiss JL: Clinical implications of imipramine plasma levels for depressive illness. *Arch. Gen. Psychiatry 34:*197–204, 1977.
7. Kane J, Rifkin A, Quitkin F, Klein DF: Antidepressant drug blood levels, pharmacokinetics and clinical outcome. In: Klein DF, Gittelman-Klein R (eds) *Progress in Psychiatric Drug Treatment.* Vol. 2. New York, Brunner/Mazel, 1976.
8. Fink M: Electroconvulsive therapy—a reevaluation. *Arch. Gen. Psychiatry,* 1977 (in press).
9. Glassman A, Kantor S, Shostak M: Depression, delusions and drug response. *Am. J. Psychiatry 132:*716–719, 1975.

8

Prevention of Recurrent Affective Disorder

JONATHAN O. COLE

Prophylactic pharmacotherapy for affective disorders is an idea whose time has really come. In the past year, two excellent reviews of the literature on the subject appeared in major psychiatric journals.[1,2] There are now available also two books of technical papers on basic and clinical aspects of lithium as a drug and as a treatment.[3,4] The latter book is primarily British in origin; both contain chapters on a variety of subjects by a wide range of authors.

Although public interest in lithium has been aroused by television shows and articles in the lay press for several years, the recent publication of books aimed at intelligent laymen by Kline[5] and by Fieve[6] has aroused a new wave of popular interest in the drug prophylaxis of recurrent affective disorders and has caused many individuals who have never before seen a psychiatrist to realize that a treatment may exist for their periodic mood swings. I have personally seen at least ten patients over the last few years whose mood swings, though distressing to the individual when depressed and sometimes to the family when hypomanic, nevertheless have never been disabling and had never required psychiatric hospitalization or even consultation. Since most of these patients' mood changes appeared to be "endogenous," I have inferred that manic-depressive disease exists in mild, as well as severe, forms.

The existence of a therapy for an illness appears both to uncover mild variants of the illness and to increase the likelihood that patients showing some features of the disease will receive the treatable condition as a primary diagnosis. At McLean and elsewhere, I have noted a growing tendency to diagnose mania rather than schizophrenic excitement whenever possible.

JONATHAN O. COLE • McLean Hospital, Belmont, Massachusetts.

It is interesting that the emergence of treatments for recurrent depression and/or mania have been accompanied by changes in diagnostic criteria and terminology which tend to shift American diagnosis away from overdiagnosing schizophrenia[7] and toward a nomenclature which emphasizes the longitudinal course of illness.The terms *unipolar* and *bipolar* affective disorder are now widely used[8] and appear to be more relevant for the study of potentially prophylactic therapies than older ways of describing and classifying depressions. (See Chapter 1 by Schatzberg.)

Evidence may be emerging that unipolar and bipolar depressions differ in their response to tricyclic drugs; imipramine appears to be effective in unipolar depressives with low MHPG excretion and amitriptyline in unipolar depressives with high MHPG excretion.[9] Schildkraut and others have demonstrated that bipolar depressives tend to demonstrate low MHPG excretion, and, by extension, they may be more responsive to treatment with imipramine. (See Chapter 3 by Schildkraut et al.)

All this interest relevant to the drug prophylaxis of affective illness arose at the same time that a substantial body of evidence was emerging that attested to the value of prophylactic antipsychotic drug therapy in averting relapse in schizophrenic patients.[10,11]

There are recurring problems in considering prophylactic or maintenance therapy for either affective illness or schizophrenia. Is a future episode of illness being averted completely by the drug therapy? Are its manifestations merely being reduced by the drug treatment? Or has the active illness always been present underneath a continuing active therapy? For the purposes of this discussion, these distinctions are deemed to be of minor importance. However, those controlled studies of maintenance drug therapy in either affective illness or schizophrenia which transfer stabilized drug-treated patients in remission to placebo generally note the timing of the observed acute relapses to be scattered over months or even years. If the drugs had been only suppressing ongoing episodes of illness, relapses would probably have clustered in the first few days or weeks on placebo.

THE DEVELOPMENT OF LITHIUM PROPHYLAXIS

It is fascinating to observe, retrospectively, the scientific–clinical resistance to accepting the idea of a prophylactic drug. Baastrup and

Schou's[12] article reported that both bipolar and unipolar patients on lithium, when compared to their prelithium frequency of affective episodes, showed an 80% decrease in time spent in serious illness and a shift in frequency of attacks from one every eight months to one every five to seven years. This was the first of a number of "mirror-image" studies in which patients with frequent attacks of unipolar or bipolar illness had their episodes for two to five years prelithium; this was compared with patients' courses for two or more years after they were given lithium. Such studies are generally comparable in outcome to the Baastrup and Schou report. Nevertheless, Blackwell and Shepard[13] in England picked a number of holes in the original design of the study and advanced the proposition that in most patients recurrent affective illnesses get less frequent over time. I was personally willing to accept the Baastrup–Schou study as evidence that a powerful drug effect had been demonstrated that simply could not be all bias or placebo effect; subsequent studies have proved Schou to be right and Shepard to be wrong, but one wonders why the initial report was attacked so vigorously.

The Baastrup–Schou study typifies the way that maintenance or prophylactic treatments have to be discovered at our present empirical level of knowledge in clinical psychopharmacology. A treatment works in an acute illness. Patients who have been sick with the same illness are kept on the drug once they are well again. If many of them have no recurrences or infrequent recurrences, the clinician–investigator begins to suspect that illnesses are being averted or substantially reduced in severity. It takes a good deal longer for controlled studies of prophylactic efficacy to be conceived and carried out. The next phase, with lithium, was the execution of drug withdrawal studies in which patients already successfully maintained on lithium were randomly assigned to further lithium or to placebo, double blind. The earliest Baastrup–Schou[14] prospective controlled study took patients already established at least one year on lithium—obviously a group of presumed lithium responders—while more recent discontinuation studies[15,16] randomly assigned patients to lithium and placebo after only a brief stabilization period on lithium. Only one[17] of the eight published controlled studies[18–21] comparing lithium and placebo as maintenance therapies in recurrent bipolar affective disorder actually randomized all patients from the beginning.

Any way you look at this imposing data mass from the eight studies, the results are strikingly positive. Davis,[1] in his recent review, has gone to the trouble of calculating an overall significance level pooling all the data and attests that the probability that such a result could be obtained by chance is not one in a thousand ($p = .001$) but one chance in 10^{86}, a number for which I know no name.

Quitkin, Rifkin, and Klein[2] detect one flaw in the currently available data. The available controlled studies which clearly identify the bipolar patients studied and the type of relapses observed (manic or depressive[14,15,16,19,20] provided clear evidence that lithium reduces significantly the number of manic relapses, but the evidence supporting a parallel reduction in depressive relapses is a good deal weaker. This is partly due to the lower incidence of depressive than manic relapses on placebo (68% versus 13%) in these studies and partly due to the majority of the bipolar patients[15] being selected in the manic phase and having a preponderence of manic relapses. Prien's smaller sample of bipolar patients selected while depressed[16] had predominantly depressive relapses. Nevertheless, the overall potency of lithium in preventing affective relapses as a group is still very impressive.

Since acute lithium therapy is clearly effective only in mania—its efficacy in depression being still highly controversial—it is fascinating to look at the pooled data from placebo-controlled studies of lithium prophylaxis, separating bipolar from unipolar patients. As can be seen from Tables I and II, the two types of affective disorder respond in essentially the same manner and clearly do far better on lithium than on placebo.

Therefore, there is excellent evidence that lithium is markedly better than inert placebo in both unipolar and bipolar recurrent affective disorders.

ANTIDEPRESSANTS

Lithium is the only available therapy conclusively shown to prevent recurrent manic episodes. No one has even seriously studied the chronic maintenance use of antipsychotic drugs, a possible alternate approach. Following bipolar patients closely, ready to intervene rapidly with antidepressants when depression begins and with haloperidol when hypomania emerges, is probably done clinically but has not been studied at all. This procedure may not be free of problems; I have recently wondered if I were not creating an iatrogenic three-week cycle in a

TABLE I. POOLED DATA FROM CONTROLLED STUDIES—LITHIUM VS. PLACEBO

	Bipolar patients	
	Total	Relapsed
Placebo	172	147 (85%)
Lithium	173	55 (32%)

bipolar patient by giving a high dose of imipramine whenever the patient became depressed, only to find him suddenly manic three weeks later. Suppressing the mania with haloperidol then leads to depression in about two weeks. Decreasing the vigor of my psychopharmacological interventions seems to have improved matters.

For unipolar patients, however, five controlled studies[16,22–25] have shown very nicely the ability of tricyclic antidepressants to prevent relapses or recurrences of depression. Table III shows the overall efficacy figures. The relapse rate on placebo in these studies is lower than in the comparable lithium–placebo studies (44% vs. 71%), probably because the lithium study patients were all selected as having had two to four previous episodes in the past two to three years, whereas the studies of prophylactic effect of antidepressant drugs more commonly picked a miscellaneous group of depressed patients with no stipulation as to the frequency or even the existence of previous episodes.

The Prien VA–NIMH study[16] is the only one directly comparing depressed patients randomly assigned to lithium, imipramine, and placebo. In this study the prophylactic efficacy of the two drugs was essentially identical. In Prien's small sample of bipolar patients ran-

TABLE II. POOLED DATA FROM CONTROLLED STUDIES—LITHIUM VS. PLACEBO

	Unipolar patients	
	Total	Relapsed
Placebo	69	49 (71%)
Lithium	76	20 (26%)

TABLE III. POOLED DATA FROM CONTROLLED STUDIES—TRICYCLICS VS. PLACEBO OR DIAZEPAM

	Total	Relapsed
Placebo	202	107 (52%)
Tricyclics	162	44 (27%)

domly assigned to imipramine, two-thirds experienced manic episodes as compared with one-third of the placebo group and one-ninth of the lithium group. Although Prien feels that this aspect of the study needs to be redone in a larger sample, I am personally satisfied that maintenance therapy with tricyclic antidepressants alone in a mania-prone patient is risky. The efficacy of combination therapy with both antidepressants and lithium in bipolar patients has never been seriously studied, although the combination must be widely used clinically by now.

MAINTENANCE DRUG THERAPY VS. PSYCHOTHERAPY

One excellent study has been carried out by Klerman[26] comparing amitriptyline, psychotherapy, and the combination in depressed patients. The results are clear and reasonable: the drug is better than placebo in reducing depressive symptoms while psychotherapy is better than minimal in improving social adjustment. The two treatments seem to work on different aspects of a patient's problems.

On a much less rigorous basis, it is my general clinical impression that many patients with recurrent affective disorders have a variety of marital and personal problems that are troublesome, regardless of whether the affective episodes are adequately controlled. Some of these are surely the secondary effects of years of disrupted existence, while others might have been present in any event; in either case, psychotherapy is often either desirable or necessary.

PROBLEMS IN MAINTENANCE DRUG THERAPY

When one reads positive articles on maintenance drug therapy, the overall impression can be mildly euphoric. The wonderful new drugs will solve all problems! Unfortunately, this is not always the whole story.

Some patients simply do not tolerate lithium well. Tremor of the hands can be a major handicap to some. Even propanolol (10–40 mg up to four times a day) does not always suppress the tremor. Some patients have nausea secondary to stomach irritation. Some gain weight and cannot tolerate the change in their body image. Some feel "strange" or get mild thinking difficulty or impairment of coordination on lithium. Although various stratagems—rearranging dosage schedule or settling for a potentially inadequate maintenance blood level—are possible, a few patients simply cannot tolerate lithium from the beginning.

Later in therapy, some develop a diabetes insipidus-like syndrome of polyurea and polydipsia which requires stopping the drug. Rare patients get enlarged thyroid glands.

However, most patients do tolerate lithium well, and it seems to mix with a variety of other psychiatric and nonpsychiatric drugs without event. In my experience, even thiazide diuretics can occasionally be added cautiously to lithium without dire effects, although lithium levels should be carefully followed in such situations.

Most of the contraindications to lithium therapy listed in the FDA's package insert seem only relative or dubious. Patients with brain damage or compensated heart disease seem to tolerate the drug well. The availability of blood level determinations makes monitoring of lithium a more secure and rational procedure than is the case with most drugs.

The more serious problem with maintenance lithium therapy is ineffectiveness. The Prien study[15] showed a 50% relapse rate in lithium-treated bipolar patients. The other controlled studies, however, have an average lithium relapse rate of only 14%, and Prien's data suggest that a higher maintenance blood lithium level (over 0.8 milliequivalents per liter) was associated with greater stability of mood. Therefore, the earlier impression that 0.5 or 0.6 was an adequate blood level may simply have been wrong. Some recurrences of mania or depression in lithium-maintained patients are, of course, due to patients' stopping their medication for various reasons. One problematic reason is that patients either miss their prior euphoric episodes or find that their past successful functioning in the arts or business only was possible when "high." Some patients with frequent mood swings find lithium prevents "highs" but not "lows" and feel cheated. There is also evidence that patients plagued by frequent, intense shifts in mood (rapid cyclers) are particularly unlikely to respond to lithium, and these are often the patients who seem to need stabilization the most urgently.

Maintenance treatment with tricyclic antidepressants is not trouble-free either. Weight gain is again a problem. Anticholinergic effects—dry mouth, blurred vision, urinary problems—are sometimes persistent and unpleasant. Lowered dose or use of peripheral cholinergic drugs (e.g., urecholine, bethanechol chloride, 25 mg, t.i.d.)[27] can sometimes solve this problem. Impotence is not helped by urecholine and can be a real curse. The issue of drug-induced changes in the electrocardiogram is currently unresolved. Such changes are worrisome. At present, it is impossible to know whether or not such changes are causally related to serious cardiac events in older patients. Some patients on tricyclics may also experience mild memory or thinking disorders, probably secondary to the central anticholinergic effects of these drugs. And there is the possibility of precipitating a manic or other psychotic episode, even in patients without prior histories of mania.

FUTURE PROSPECTS

Given that many, but by no means all, patients with bipolar or unipolar recurrent affective disorders can have their future episodes totally prevented or markedly alleviated by lithium or tricyclic antidepressants, or both, what will the future bring for those patients not presently being helped?

For some present patients, an increase in the maintenance lithium or antidepressant level may help. Occasionally, one finds a patient who simply has forgotten the rule that lithium blood levels should be taken twelve hours after the last dose and has been taking his lithium two hours before his blood is drawn, leading to inadequate dose titration.

There is a little suggestive evidence that monitoring blood cell lithium rather than plasma lithium might provide a better index of brain lithium[28] and be a better basis for setting a stable prophylactic dose. This technique is just being started at a number of institutions.

For patients on maintenance antidepressants, the newer methods for measuring blood levels should be used in the monitoring of patients during maintenance therapy. The single available relevant paper[29] reported that at least 17% of a group of 150 depressed outpatients had grossly inadequate tricyclic blood levels and another 14% probably had excessive blood levels. Unfortunately, we are not yet fully able to interpret the blood levels obtained from patients on tricyclics. Some, but not all, studies suggest[30] that there is a therapeutic window for nortriptyline with patients with higher levels being overtreated and those with lower levels being undertreated. Glassman[31] has recently shown that depressed patients with combined imipramine–desmethyl imipramine levels of less than approximately 180 ng also do not respond clinically. These blood-level methods seem useful to have available and can help suggest in which direction to alter dosage in patients who are not doing well on maintenance tricyclic therapy.

Techniques of clinical management of patients with recurrent affective disorders are also in flux. They often do not need intensive psychotherapy but do need some level of regular monitoring of affective state and drug level. For some, a medication group of drug maintenance patients—or for patients and their spouses—may be a good solution. For others, some mixture of regular brief telephone contacts with monthly or bimonthly office visits may be more suitable.

Some patients will be steadily euthymic on lithium alone. Others require short-term medication with other drugs to correct for residual mood swings. Maintenance therapy logistics are therefore potentially quite different from those required by short-term crisis intervention or psychotherapy or even psychoanalysis.

In summary, lithium carbonate is evidently a very useful prophylactic therapy in many unipolar and bipolar manic-depressive patients. Tricyclic antidepressants are about as useful in unipolar patients. Hopefully, improved methods for monitoring body levels of both types of drug and better systems for assuring that patients adhere to adequate maintenance regimens will increase the general utility of these unique advances in the treatment and prevention of affective disorders.

REFERENCES

1. Davis J: Overview: Maintenance therapy in psychiatry: II Affective disorders. *Am. J. Psychiatry 133:*1–13, 1976.
2. Quitkin F, Rifkin A, Klein DF: Prophylaxis of affective disorders. *Arch. Gen. Psychiatry* 33:337–341, 1976.
3. Gershon S, Shopsin B (eds) *Lithium.* New York, Plenum Press, 1973.
4. Johnson FN (ed) *Lithium Research and Therapy.* London, Academic Press, 1975.
5. Kline N: *From Sad to Glad.* New York, Putnam, 1974.

6. Fieve RR: *Moodswing, The Third Revolution in Psychiatry*. New York, William Morrow, 1975.
7. Gurland B, Fleiss J, Cooper J, Kendall R, Simon R: Cross-national study of diagnosis of the mental disorders. *Am. J. Psychiatry 125,* Supplement to No. 10:30–39, 1969.
8. Robins E, Guze S: Classification of affective disorders. In: Williams T, Katz M, Shield J (eds) *Recent Advances in the Psychobiology of the Depressive Illnesses, USDHEW Publication 70-9053,* p. 283–293. Washington, GPO, 1972.
9. Backmann H, Goodwin FK: Antidepressant response to tricyclics and urinary MHPG in unipolar patients. *Arch. Gen. Psychiatry 32:*17–21, 1975.
10. Davis, JM: Maintenance therapy in psychiatry: I. Schizophrenia. *Am. J. Psychiatry 132:*1237–1245, 1975.
11. Gardos G, Cole JO: Maintenance antipsychotic therapy: Is the cure worse than the disease? *Am. J. Psychiatry 133:*32–36, 1976.
12. Baastrup P, Schou M: Lithium as a prophylactic agent against recurrent depressions and manic-depressive psychosis. *Arch. Gen. Psychiatry 16:*162–172, 1967.
13. Blackwell B, Shepard M: Prophylactic lithium: Another therapeutic myth? An examination of evidence to date. *Lancet 1:*968–971, 1968.
14. Baastrup P, Poulsen K, Schou M et al.: Prophylactic lithium: Double-blind discontinuation in manic-depressive and recurrent-depressive disorders. *Lancet 2:*326–330, 1970.
15. Prien R, Caffey E, Klett CJ: Prophylactic efficacy of lithium carbonate in manic-depressive illness. *Arch. Gen. Psychiatry 28:*337–341, 1973.
16. Prien R, Klett CJ, Caffey E: Lithium carbonate and imipramine in the prevention of affective disorders. *Arch. Gen. Psychiatry 29:*420–425, 1973.
17. Coppen A, Noguera R, Bailey J et al.: Prophylactic lithium in affective disorders. *Lancet 2:*275–279, 1971.
18. Melia PI: Prophylactic lithium: A double-blind trial in recurrent affective disorders. *Br. J. Psychiatry 116:*621–624, 1970.
19. Stallone F, Shelley E, Mendlewica J et al.: The use of lithium in affective disorders. III. A double-blind study of prophylaxis in bipolar illness. *Am. J. Psychiatry 130:*1006–1010, 1973.
20. Cundall RL, Brooks PW, Murray LG: A controlled evaluation of lithium prophylaxis in affective disorders. *Psychol. Med. 2:*308–311, 1972.
21. Hullen RP, McDonald R, Allsopp MNE: Prophylactic lithium in recurrent affective disorders. *Lancet 1:*1044–1046, 1972.
22. Seager CP, Bird RL: Imipramine with electrical treatment in depression: A controlled trial. *J. Ment. Sci. 108:*704–707, 1962.
23. Kay DWK, Fahy T, Garside RF: A seven-month double-blind trial of amitriptyline and diazepam in ECT-treated depressed patients. *Br. J. Psychiatry 117:*667–671, 1970.
24. Mindman RHS, Howland D, Shepard M: An evaluation of continuation therapy with tricyclic antidepressants in depressive illness. *Psychol. Med. 3:*5–17, 1973.
25. Klerman GL, DiMascio A, Weissman M et al.: Treatment of depression by drugs and psychotherapy. *Am. J. Psychiatry 131:*186–191, 1974.
26. Klerman GL: Combining drugs and psychotherapy in the treatment of depression. In: Greenblatt M (ed) *Drugs in Combination with Other Therapies.* New York, Grune and Stratton, 1975.
27. Everett HC: The use of bethanechol chloride with tricyclic antidepressants. *Am. J. Psychiatry 132:*1202–1203, 1975.
28. Mendels J, Frazer A: Intracellular lithium concentration and clinical response: Towards a membrane theory of depression. *J. Psychiat. Res. 10:*9–19, 1973.
29. Biggs J, Chang S, Sherman W, Holland W: Measurement of tricyclic antidepressant levels in an out-patient clinic. *J. Nerv. Ment. Dis. 162:*46–51, 1976.

30. Kane J, Rifkin A, Quitkin F, Klein DF: Antidepressant drug blood levels, pharmacokinetics and clinical outcome. In: Klein DF, Gittelman-Klein K (eds) *Progress in Psychiatric Drug Treatment,* Vol. II, pp. 136–158. New York, Brunner/Mazel, 1976.
31. Glassman A, Perel J: Tricyclic blood levels and clinical outcome. In: Lipton M, DiMascio A, Killam K (eds) *A Generation of Progress in Psychopharmacology*. New York, Raven Press, 1977.

9

Psychoanalytic Contribution to a Theory of Depression

PHILLIP L. ISENBERG and ALAN F. SCHATZBERG

Recent advances in biological research of depression may lead practitioners to adopt a stance that some depressions are biologically caused, whereas others are psychologically determined. Some may go so far as to argue that the classic endogenous or autonomous depression is due solely to biochemical or biological causes, whereas the neurotic depressive disorder is due entirely to psychological factors. Such an assumption would be simplistic, since neurotic disorders have physiologic symptoms (e.g., sleep disturbance, tachycardia, etc.) and patients may experience endogenous depressions after a specific loss, disappointment, or psychological injury. Recently, Akiskal and McKinney[1] have attempted to synthesize various psychodynamic, neurochemical, and neurophysiological theories in an effort to understand depressive disorders. Although we advocate incorporating a psychoanalytic viewpoint to such an approach, we feel this is difficult, since a unified, comprehensive, and precise psychoanalytic theory of depression has not fully emerged. Rather, there has been a tendency within psychoanalysis for discrete theoretical approaches to be applied to a host of diagnostic categories (including schizophrenia, neuroses, borderline states, and several types of depression), thus obscuring crucial diagnostic differentiation. Also, although many psychoanalytic theories exist, few have attempted to differentiate among the many subtypes of depressive disorders. This difficulty reflects a more general problem in the classification of psychiatric disorders, including depression. In addition, there has existed a limited differentiation in psychoanalytic theory

PHILLIP L. ISENBERG and ALAN F. SCHATZBERG • Department of Psychiatry, Harvard Medical School, Boston, Massachusetts, and McLean Hospital, Belmont, Massachusetts.

between the dynamics of a depressive episode and those psychological factors (generally early developmental deficits) which may predispose individuals. Moreover, the literature has often failed to distinguish between depressive affect and/or mood and depressive illness. All of these factors have hampered efforts at developing a synthesized psychoanalytic theory of depression.

The psychoanalytic literature on depressive disorders has dealt mainly with clinical description and theory rather than with nosology and treatment. Although the early papers of Abraham[2] and Freud[3] show an astute and far-reaching grasp of the psychodynamics underlying depressive disorders, a clear application of their theories to therapy and nosology was lacking, a state of affairs noted by Freud himself. It is our own belief that nosology, psychodynamic theory, and treatment (both psychotherapeutic and psychopharmacologic) must go hand in hand in a comprehensive investigation of psychopathology. In recent years, advances in psychopharmacology, biology, and computer analysis have led to progress in nosology and to improved clinical care. Over time, such advances may also support the development of a more specific and comprehensive analytic theory, which could be productively applied to the various subtypes of depressions.

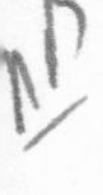

In this chapter we shall review critically some psychoanalytic approaches to depressive disorders. Emphasis will be placed on highlighting how the major themes may be applied and synthesized to provide an approach to both understanding and treating depressive disorders, particularly unipolar endogenous depression. We shall also attempt to trace the psychological development of a clear-cut endogenous or autonomous state, integrating psychodynamics, somatic symptoms, cognitive distortions, and mood disturbances. This review is offered with the hope that it will both provide a practical guide to the dynamics of depression and support further study of classification and psychodynamic theory.

REVIEW OF THE LITERATURE

For the purpose of this paper we have divided psychoanalytic theory into four major approaches: libidinal, ego psychological, object relations, and cognitive. Of course, psychoanalytic approaches can be looked at in different ways, of which this organization is but one. Further, because of a limitation in space, we have included only representative works. The reader is referred elsewhere for a more detailed review of the literature.[4–6]

Libidinal Approach

Early psychoanalytic theories emphasized libidinal drives and psychosexual development. Such writings were often colored with vivid imagery and emphasis on energy systems. Abraham, the greatest contributor to a libidinal psychoanalytic approach, was first to postulate orality and ambivalence as the key factors in the etiology of depression. In 1911, he proposed that depressed manic-depressive patients mourn their lost capacity to love.[2] Regressing to a level of oral fixation in which they desire to incorporate the love object, their affects are colored by a devouring rage and hostility. "He behaves as though the complete abstention of food alone could keep him from carrying out his repressed impulses, but at the same time he threatens himself with that punishment which alone is fitting for his unconscious cannibalistic drives—death by starvation." In 1924, he elaborated upon this theory and postulated that oral eroticism predisposes individuals to depressive illness.[7] Oral fixation, the result of repeated disappointments in the subject's relationship with mother, leads to intensely ambivalent adult relationships. When adult love relationships fail, anger results, which, when introjected, leads to the lowered self-esteem seen in depressed patients.

Building on Abraham's early work, Freud (*In Mourning and Melancholia,* 1917) emphasized the key role of lowered self-esteem, which occurred in melancholia (depression) but not in mourning.[3] This differentiation between mourning and melancholia has become a leitmotif of analytic theory and nosology. In melancholia, the subject responds with rage to a real or perceived loss and directs the rage first against the object and eventually against the self after the fateful incorporation of the object. "So we find the key to the clinical pictures: we perceive that the self-reproaches are reproaches against the loved object which has been shifted away from it onto the patient's own ego." The inability to continue to direct the anger toward the object is explained on the basis of regression to an oral–narcissistic stage of development, consistent with the tendency to incorporate the object following loss. Freud felt such regression was common in individuals whose previous relationships were primarily narcissistic, but this factor was neither clearly defined nor elaborated.

Regarding nosological discrimination, both Freud and Abraham wrote ostensibly on manic-depressive psychosis. Their emphasis, however, was on the depressive episode with an attempt to gear their theories to address manic states as well, albeit as a seeming afterthought. Perhaps their ostensible writings on manic-depressive illness reflected the Kraepelinian notion that all depressions were variants of manic-depressive illness (see Chapter 1 by Schatzberg). Both theories may be viewed as "pyramidal" in that a recent loss has great repercussions, since early developmental tasks were not mastered. For Abraham, the early developmental task is a resolution of oral dependency; for Freud, it is a maturation beyond a narcissistic object choice.

The central importance of self-esteem and self-criticism in *Mourning and Melancholia* led to the formulation of a theory of the superego which Rado[8,9] and other psychoanalytic writers have applied and stressed in understanding and treating depressive disorders. Rado emphasized that depressives rely on external support for narcissistic supplies to maintain their self-esteem. When depressives lose their nurturing objects, they respond with rage. This rage is viewed intrapsychically as one partial introject of the lost object (conceived of as situated within the superego) railing against another partial introject of the same object (situated within the ego of the patient). By postulating the unique concept of the double introject, Rado attempted to combine the newer structural theory (involving ego and superego functions) with the earlier theories as seen in *Mourning and Melancholia.* Depression was viewed as an intrapsychic process of expiation and a plea for forgiveness. It is our belief that this theory is often quite confusing and difficult to apply to understanding and treating the depressed patient, though Jacobson arrived at a similar construction from a different pathway.

Ego-Psychological Theory

As psychoanalytic theory developed, theorists began to study general ego functions, their development, and their role in psychiatric disorders. Thus, the emphasis began to move away from libido theory. Interestingly, these writings are often less colored with vivid imagery than are earlier papers. At any rate, although the overall emphasis changed, nosological problems persisted. Bibring,[10] the major contributor to understanding the common ego mechanisms underlying depression, postulated that depressives responded to their own perceived failure to fulfill their ego ideal aspirations and became depressed as a result of the realization of this failure. Oral fixation was not vital to his theory, although it could be a common predisposing feature or mechanism of recovery. The goals to be strong and superior, or to be good, loving, and nonaggressive, or to be appreciated and worthy, all represented aspirations in turn related to specific libidinal levels of development. Although Bibring, and Zetzel[11] after him, attempted to develop an exclusively ego-psychological theory, his effort was rooted in earlier libido theory. In addition, Bibring attempted to construct a parallel theory for depression to Freud's theory of signal anxiety in *Inhibitions, Symptoms and Anxiety.*[12] Nevertheless, a basic understanding of affects was not yet adequate to clarify depressive disorders with these conceptual tools.

Rubinfine criticized Bibring's thesis, feeling it did not account for why some individuals are prone to depressive illness and others not.[13] Using object relations theory, he proposed that a depressive predisposition was the result of the subject's "fixation to a state of narcissistic unity with the mother." He noted that when, in his early years, the subject may have been faced with repetitive frustrating "rather than gratifying experiences . . . there is a premature development of individuation-separation (Mahler)." In addition, he noted that "there is a premature differentiation of the aggressive drive." Unable to deal with this rage, the infant regressed to an earlier symbiotic stage of development. Frustration, rage, and the internalization of the bad object are essential in his eyes for understanding depression. Like Abraham, Rubinfine proposed that this constellation of events reappears after disappointments in adult love relationships. He suggested Bibring's theory of the mechanism of depression on the other hand was a general one, applicable to those human situations in which depressive affect is experienced. He differentiated between depressive illness and depressive affect as a signal and elaborated the theoretical basis for understanding each.

Object Relations Theory

In recent years, great emphasis has been placed on the nature of individuals' object relations, their internal representations, and their importance to general psychological functioning and psychopathology. Much of this emphasis is based on principles first put forth by Melanie Klein. Depression has a unique meaning in Kleinian theory and is related to specific developmental tasks which she postulated must be partially resolved in early infancy to obtain any psychic equilibrium. More specifically, the paranoid–schizoid and depressive positions represent key psychological tasks of infancy.[14,15] Kleinian theory increasingly has had application in the understanding and treatment of psychotic and borderline states. The theory suggests that depressive disorders are basically rooted in disturbances in the first year of life. A basic assumption of this view is that there is a psychotic core to all patients, an assumption which has met with great criticism. In the paranoid–schizoid position, anxiety regarding the death instinct is defended against by splitting of objects into good and bad parts. Projective identification is used in dealing with the bad "persecutory objects." Later, in the depressive position, the infant must deal with the fear of losing the important, "good" object by virtue of its anger towards the object through mastery of this rage. The successful negotiation of this stage is vital to one's immunity from subsequent serious depressions. In later life, losses of important objects reactivate the depressive position with its specific set of feelings; namely, ambivalence, rage, and fear of separation. "Just as the young child passing through the depressive position is struggling, in his unconscious mind, with the task of establishing and integrating his inner world, so the mourner goes through the pain of re-establishing and re-integrating it."[15] Klein notes that in the depressive position the infant experiences the "good mother" to some degree, and these internalized good objects can be relied upon when, and if, a key object is lost in later life. This, coupled with outside support, enables the mourner to avoid a depressive illness.

Winnicott, relying heavily on the work of Klein, also emphasized the depressive position.[16] He believed that in this stage the infant must learn to reconcile the two images of the mother, the loving "good object" and the withholding "bad" one, the counterparts of frustrating and gratifying exchanges with the mother. The attempt to bring these two objects together engenders guilt and tension in the child. Over time, however, he must deal with his rage and integrate the two images in order to develop the capacity for whole object relations. Again, following Klein, he notes that the loss of an object in later adult life results in depression if the depressive position has not been successfully negotiated in infancy.

> Mourning means that the object loss has been magically introjected (as Freud showed); it is there subjected to hate. I suppose to mean that it is allowed contact with internal persecutory elements. Incidentally, the inner world balance of forces is upset by this, so that the persecutory elements are increased and the benign or supportive forces are weakened. There is a danger situation, and the defensive mechanism of an overall deadening produces depression. The depression is a healing mechanism; it covers the battleground with a mist, allowing for a sorting out at a reduced rate, giving time for all possible defenses to be brought into play, and for a working through, so that eventually there can be a spontaneous recovery.[16]

In the individual who has successfully negotiated the depressive position in infancy, loss of an object results in grief and not depression as memories of the good object support the individual's coping mechanisms. "Love of the internal representation of an external object lost can lessen the hate of the introjected love object which loss entails. In these and other ways mourning is experienced and worked through, and grief can be felt as such." Again one hears the familiar theme of mourning or melancholia.

One clinical study which restricted itself to a specific type of depression was that of Cohen et al.[17] Investigating a group of manic-depressive patients and their families, they proposed a set of common variables and dynamics. Manic-depressives were felt to be fixated in their development at a point earlier than neurotics but later than schizophrenics. Hence, the maturity of their object relations was also felt to be intermediate. These investigators suggested, as did Klein, Winnicott, and others, that manic-depressive patients split the maternal representation into good and bad images, which they cannot integrate. Instead, they learn to deal with objects only via manipulation. Family dynamics which contributed to this style included an isolation of the family from its surrounding social network and an expectation that the patient will perform some extraordinary task and save the family from their collective problems. Such attitudes are paradoxically mixed with envy. In response, the patient tends to undersell himself to others, to promote others, and to please authority figures to achieve acceptance. Depression occurs when he is faced with the realization that he, himself, will not be fulfilled in the real world as a result of this style of coping. Although this study is often cited, it is our belief that further, more systematic study is required to validate it.

Utilizing her basic concepts on individuation/separation, Mahler developed a theory on the genesis of depressive *affects*.[18] However, the relationship between depressive affects and illnesses is not clear in her work. Further, it is unclear whether she is addressing "primitive" characterologic disease in which depression is but one, albeit important, symptom or whether she is describing an endogenous depressive disorder. In studying infantile psychoses and early development, she emphasized that the mastery of separation must be resolved in infancy in order to achieve later psychic health. One major aspect of separation is an inevitable developmental conflict around symbiotic omnipotence. To separate means that the child must acknowledge that neither he nor the parent is omnipotent. At times, the child attempts to adhere to a oneness with his parents such that the acknowledgement of separation leaves him with feelings of futility, ambivalence, and hostile dependency. Failure to resolve this conflict predisposes the individual to later depressive illness. As Mahler has stated[18]:

> I believe that the collapse of the child's belief in his own omnipotence, with his uncertainty about the emotional availability of the parents, creates the so-called "hostile dependency" upon and ambivalence towards the parents. This ambivalence seems to call for the early pathological defense mechanisms of splitting the good and bad mother images and of turning aggression against the self; these result in a feeling of helplessness, which, as Bibring (1953) has emphasized, creates the basic depressive affect. These libidino–economic circumstances may become the basis for responding habitually with negative mood swings.

Also, she states, "The two pillars of early infantile well-being and self-esteem are the child's belief in his own omnipotence and his belief in the parents' omnipotence, of which he partakes; these beliefs can be replaced only gradually by a realistic recognition of, belief in, and enjoyment of his individual autonomy and the development of object constancy (Hartmann, 1952)."

In her extended studies of depression, Jacobson elaborated a comprehensive theory which relies on modern ego psychology.[19] After clarifying the development of self and object representations and the formation of ego ideal and superego, she carefully outlined the pathological processes which can lead to a lowered self-esteem, the final common pathway to depressive illness. More specifically, she emphasized an unattainable ego ideal, a fiercely harsh superego, and an ego apparatus which cannot achieve adequately as those convergent forces which lead to depressive illness. In his premorbid state, the subject is markedly dependent and thus relies on the strength, power, and value of his love object, using denial as a mechanism to maintain this state of affairs intrapsychically, ignoring the real defects in the object.

This unbalanced relationship, based on unrealistic idealization, leads to inevitable disappointment and frustration with states of tension that produce symptom formation in the vulnerable personality of the depressive. This pattern can be of neurotic or psychotic proportions. With massive frustration, narcissistic regression, or fusion of self and object representations, it produces a psychotic picture. This description of fusion restates more precisely Freud's famous description that "the shadow of the object falls upon the ego." In addition, Jacobson, using the terminology of self and object representations and their fusion, clarifies the essential process first suggested by Freud as the main line of development in depressive illness: that the narcissistic object relationship regresses in the illness proper to a narcissistic identification. Jacobson's work is a helpful guide in the psychotherapy of depressive patients, since she describes in detail the several problems which often arise in therapy—massive dependency, provocative masochistic gestures, and narcissistic withdrawal.

To summarize, modern psychoanalytic approaches have relied primarily on the concept of development of object relations. The infant is seen as needing to resolve fundamental danger situations sequentially to assure maturation and differentiation consistent with adult emotional capabilities. Depressive disorders, therefore, are seen as disturbances secondary to the failure to resolve a basic ambivalence with the nurturing mother (i.e., failure to resolve the depressive position), or a failure to resolve infantile omnipotence (Mahler), or failure to establish well-defined self and object representations, mature ideals, and a loving superego (Jacobson). In the premorbid period this failure is obscured by reliance on such primitive defenses as denial, introjection, projection, and avoidance. There is, nevertheless, some confusion between the dynamics of a characterologically predisposed individual and the dynamics of an isolated depressive episode, including both the illness phase and recovery phase.

Cognitive Theory

Beck has extended the psychiatric theory of depression as an affective disturbance by emphasizing a central thought disorder.[20] In studying depressed patients, he noted several common themes: low self-regard, feeling of deprivation, exaggeration of problems, self-criticism, self-commands, and suicidal ideation. He explained these themes on the basis of a cognitive triad: (1) a negative interpretation of the subject's own experience such that he sees himself as prone to failure and commonly misreads innocuous statements made about himself as meaning that he is bad; (2) a devaluation of the self; i.e., the individual will view negatively his own experience with the world; and (3) a negative view of the future, which implies that the subject will display a pessimistic attitude built on his past experience with his world.

Beck wrote that this triad is based on more specific thought patterns in depressives: arbitrary inference, selective abstraction, overgeneralization, and magnification–minimization distortions. Arbitrary inference refers to the subject's misinterpretation of statements made to him; selective abstraction refers to focusing on extraneous details; and overgeneralization to the tendency to make global conclusions about himself on the basis of one incident. Magnification and minimization both refer to errors in evaluation which are so gross as to constitute cognitive distortions. Beck developed a therapeutic approach for the suicidal depressed patient based on these ideas (see Chapter 12). While we believe that disturbances in thinking exist in the full-blown episode, the primary or etiologic significance of a thought disorder in depression is open to debate, as is its possible variation in different types of depressive disorders. Further, recent research has raised question as to the specificity of thought disorders in psychiatric illnesses.

DISCUSSION

Overall, then, the psychoanalytic literature on depression has tended to emphasize several themes, particularly orality, early object relations, and mastery of infantile rage/omnipotence and loss in adult life. However, these themes are not unique to depressive disorders; rather, many of them have been applied by the same workers to describe several possible psychiatric illnesses, which are often not clearly specified. While overtly there are differences between libidinal and object relations theories representing as they do different periods of theory making and different emphases, similarities also exist, particularly the central roles of rage, ambivalence, and incorporation. Object relations theory has, however, explored in some detail the issues of early development, especially in regard to primitive ego states and their functions. In both theories, precipitants for a depressive episode have generally revolved around recent object loss and its relationship to early developmental problems. So strong is this trend in psychoanalysis that, even though Bibring emphasized more general ego mechanisms and the state of helplessness, his work too suggested an early fixation was essential, at least, to a state of helplessness. Rubinfine's further elaboration of Bibring's work suggested the predisposition was due to premature separation from mother and differentiation of the aggressive drive (as described by Mahler). Indeed, as a whole, the literature attempts to emphasize an essential predisposition which accounts for why some individuals become clinically depressed while others do not. Since loss of an object is often felt to rekindle an unresolved "depressive position," many of the theories (excluding Bibring's) do not take into account precipitants other than loss and their significance in the individual's psychological makeup. Interestingly, the literature has spoken of recent and early loss, ignoring the role of loss in latency or preadolescence. Recent research has indicated, however, that the kind of loss may play a major role in determining the type of depressive illness and that loss of mother prior to age eleven causes a later vulnerability to depression.[21] Although loss seems like a simple concept, in psychoanalytic theorizing it does not mean simply the unavailability of the object but rather the loss of usefulness of the object to the subject. Even the threat of loss has been implicated as a risk factor. Also, it would be more correct to say depression often has been seen as a consequence of an intolerance to accepting loss.

Further difficulty revolves around the demarcation of types of depressions. Since recent loss is often stressed and there is inadequate description of the symptomatology of the illnesses, it is unclear whether workers are addressing general grief reactions or nonendogenous depressions following a real or perceived loss rather than addressing a unipolar endogenous syndrome. Some workers, e.g., Freud and Abraham, have written about manic-depressive illness, albeit this is misleading as variations in classification between then and now may come into play. Further, a manic-depressive depressive episode may be unprecipitated by recent loss or stress (see Chapter 1 by Schatzberg). Some theorists (e.g., Klein, Winnicott, Rado) appear to be describing syndromes which represent reactions to loss, characterologic depressions, or personality disorders with a depressive overlay. However, this is not entirely clear from their work; rather, diagnosis is obscured. Finally, workers have often failed to distinguish between affect and illness. As noted previously, although Mahler's work addresses itself specifically to depressive affect, its relationship to a disease state is not fully clarified.

In the following sections, we attempt to clarify some of these issues and to develop a synthesized theory of unipolar endogenous depressions based on clinical material which will be presented.

First, it is important to separate depressive affect from illness. Depressive affect denotes a characteristic set of feelings or a disposition to feelings that are aroused in a person confronted with psychic loss, disappointment, or failure. Although this constellation of feelings is broad, feelings of helplessness and hopelessness are pivotal. They are, however, not exclusively present in depression or equivalent to it. When most writers refer to depressive affect, they also include the feelings of being let down, sadness, psychological pain resulting from a threat to one's sense of well-being, and the fear of failure of not being able to live up to one's own expectations. These depressive affects can be mobilized in people who are relatively healthy as well as those who are predisposed to severe depressive illnesses. Both Zetzel and Hartmann[22] stressed that the ability to develop conscious feelings of sadness and to acknowledge one's own and others' limitations are a prerequisite for mature emotional functioning. Thus, people can mourn some losses, suffer the absence of deserved recognitions, and bear innumerable deprivations without experiencing a clinical depression. The capacity to accept and tolerate sadness might be an indication of sufficient ego strength to be incompatible with a depressive illness. Zetzel emphasized that those people who cannot tolerate depressive affect show a special kind of vulnerability and hence a predisposition to psychopathology, not necessarily depression.

Depressive moods, Jacobson emphasized, were persistent states of depressive feelings which colored both one's perceptions and one's ability to respond adequately to experiences. Although this mood may influence most of one's experiences for days or weeks, it does not necessarily become associated with a complex of symptoms which has been characteristic of the various depressive disorders.

The depressive syndrome and/or disorders, on the other hand, are marked by a host of somatic and psychological symptoms which vary as to their intensity and type. The patient may be deeply depressed, apathetic, retarded or agitated, anorexic, anhedonic, and sleep poorly. If clearly psychotic, he may experience hallucinations and express delusions of guilt, inferiority, nihilism, and abject poverty. At a less psychotic level, thinking is characterized primarily by retardation and subjective difficulty without frank delusions. There may be preoccupation with the bodily processes, which are often slowed down; and guilt and self-depreciation are common, again without delusional conviction. The future looks hopeless, and life seems hardly worth living. Objective problems seem completely out of proportion to what the subject is, in fact, subjectively experiencing. At the mildest level of depression, he may simply have a sense that life is not interesting, and experience some social withdrawal and a lack of pleasure. Vegetative signs may vary greatly. The patient may not be aware of the depressive component to his everyday functioning and somber mood. Though psychosis and severity dimensions account for some syndrome variation, there is still debate as to the differentiation of depressive disorders on the basis of specific symptoms, outcome, or other factors.

The classification of depression has been reviewed elsewhere in this book (see Chapter 1 by Schatzberg). Of note in recent years has been the emphasis on primary depressions by some groups[23] and unipolar endogenous depressions in others.[24] Great similarities exist between the two groupings, especially the requirement of a core of vegetative symptoms in addition to lowered mood. Also, both groups have spoken of well-adjusted and adequately functioning premorbid personalities in this type of depression. It is our feeling that this is misleading, since such patients may appear on the surface well adjusted but have deep-seated psychological problems or vulnerabilities which can be quite limiting. One may wonder whether the description of preexisting psychological problems in the context of a depressive episode represents an actual difficulty or a cognitive misperception of themselves and their former world as a retrospective falsification. We favor the former view. As patients separate out preexisting issues and gain some distance from the depressive episode, we have noted an increased ability on their part to describe and acknowledge their premorbid limitations and psychological problems.

Regarding nonendogenous and secondary depressions, it appears that these may form a heterogeneous group of disorders which includes a host of neurotic and characterological problems. As such, we feel the development of a unitary theory of all depressions may be an elusive goal.

The following cases provide some clinical examples of patients with unipolar depressive disorders. They are presented to clarify both premorbid characteristics of such patients and the type of disorder to which we are referring. Indeed, as Rubinfine has noted, personality variables may predispose certain individuals to becoming depressed, implying a stepwise relationship between premorbid personality structure and depression, and he feels that evidence suggests a primarily oral personality disturbance. Others view the premorbid personality and "free periods" between attacks as either demonstrating normal healthy functioning or an obsessive–compulsive organization.[25] We believe the following case reports or excerpts demonstrate a particularly common premorbid structure which is not "normal" or healthy except as it represents a healthier state of adaptation than the episodes of depression proper, which themselves represent significant clinical regressions. It must be noted that more than one subtype of unipolar endogenous depression may exist and these cases may more accurately reflect just one subtype.

All of these patients were in their thirties or forties, engaged in work, well educated, either currently or previously married, and in long-term psychotherapy for several years. They had depressive illnesses which were well-established syndromes which responded only incompletely to environmental changes. Each patient improved with intensive psychoanalytically oriented psychotherapy and antidepressant medication.

Case Examples

A. Patient A, a woman in her thirties, gave a history of early learning disability despite superior intellectual endowment. She married soon after college but felt her husband had done her a favor by marrying her, this in spite of the fact that it was she, and not he, who was regularly employed. She experienced her needs as unnecessary complications in her life, feeling she should live by achieving and not needing anyone else. Although she appeared to function well, she had little belief in herself and felt that no one else could care for her or help her. As she became more aware of the precariousness of her marriage, which ended in divorce, her depression increased and was characterized by anorexia, weight loss, somatic anxiety, difficulty in thinking and functioning, inability to be alone, feelings of doom, and suicidal ideation. Behind a history of apparent achievement was a subjective life characterized by a lack of confidence and marked insecurity in relationships. Her relationships to her mother and older sister were poor. They were dominated by judgmental attitudes and the manipulation of feelings of guilt in each other.

B. Patient B, a man in his forties, felt a marked need for achievement and demonstrated self-sacrificing behavior in his devotion to both his profession and his family. However, he was unable to accomplish all that he had expected of himself because of the failure of the school which he directed. His devotion, concern, and love for the institution were shown to have limitations which he could not accept. He became so depressed that he lost sight of his own vital interests, left his wife and children, and lived in self-imposed seclusion. Prior to this episode of illness, he was known to be serious, hardworking, and achievement-oriented—loyal, devoted, attentive, careful, and overconcerned in his manner. Overtly, his life reflected a consistent effort at self-improvement, but there persisted a fundamental sense of emotional isolation and a lack of gratification from success or from relationships with others. He did not sense that people cared for him, although he knew he was admired for his good deeds and high standards. He feared being abandoned by others if they found him unacceptable in any way. At an early age he remembered turning away emotionally from his parents, feeling that he could never really earn their love. He felt this "loss" was the result of his hostile rejection of his parents for disappointing him.

C. Patient C presented in his late twenties because of persistent headaches and difficulty in thinking. He was aware during his depression of internal tensions and panicky moments precipitated by something as ordinary as a visit to the dentist. He had as a presenting chief complaint the delusional fear that his hair was falling out and he feared that he would be bald and unacceptable. Other symptoms included weight loss, inability to work, and hours of tearless sobbing. There was a previous history of dropping out of college because of difficulty in studying. He became depressed after his female employer, for whom he had worked for four years, died. He complained of difficulty in relating to others throughout his life and was aware that he felt alienated from people. On the other hand, he was a generous, intelligent individual who had an excellent business sense and ability to appraise people and complex situations. He was extremely sensitive to rejection and had a lifelong sense of abandonment from his parents. His parents were divorced in his childhood, and his relationship with his father was very poor. His relationship with his mother was distant and cold.

D. Patient D, a man in his thirties, came to treatment convinced that his diabetes was out of control. He was so preoccupied with his blood sugar and other somatic concerns that he had difficulty in thinking and in relating to his fiancee. Medical evaluation revealed that his diabetes was under reasonable control, although he was unable to keep to his medical regimen when depressed. It was clear that his inhibition of thinking affected his ability to communicate with people. Fear of failure, which led to indecisiveness, was so pathological that he could not work productively on assignments. He described himself as feeling then like "a mouse in a maze." His lack of initiative came from an attempt to avoid possible mistakes arising from decision-making situations. A significant conviction was that he should not accept assistance from anyone and that he should pick himself up by his own bootstraps. This attitude he attributed to lifelong patterns of relating to his mother, who insisted on his competence in everything. He typically showed a somber mood. He was restrained and humorless in his style but was a reliable, dependable, and deliberate worker as a science editor. Under tension he noted increasing rigidity in his thinking, suicidal ideation, and a fear that he could not survive.

All of these patients fulfilled symptom criteria for a diagnosis of unipolar endogenous depression (see Chapter 1 by Schatzberg). However, these examples call into question an undue emphasis on healthy premorbid personalities. They all appeared well adjusted premorbidly, the difficulties they experienced in functioning not being easily apparent to people in their environment. All of these individuals outwardly seemed successful and reasonably competent. They were warm and seemingly capable of relating in various ways to people. They were, however, in fact, deeply insecure, full of fear of failure, unconvinced of their worth whatever their accomplishments, alienated emotionally from people, yet often capable of intense identification with the suffering of others. These particular insights about their own self-image came only later in therapy when the patients had a capacity to observe themselves more objectively.

With all four patients the combined use of antidepressive medication and long-term psychotherapy was efficacious. The psychotherapeutic gains came after resolving intense conflict around rejection, promises, lack of understanding, and emotional isolation. These conflicts become the basic issues in the transference relationship and must not be sidestepped or ignored. With sufficient time and care, resolution of these issues leads to emotional growth with a better euthymic adjustment and a decreased likelihood of recurrence of depression.

A CLINICAL THEORY OF DEPRESSIVE DISORDER

How, then, can we integrate these observations and the various dynamic theories outlined above? Perhaps we should begin with commonly emphasized themes in the literature. First, ever since Freud postulated the central importance of "the loss of self-regarding feeling," psychoanalytic investigators, including Bibring, Jacobson, Sandler, and others, have repeatedly emphasized the crucial role of the fall of self-esteem in depressive disorders. Bibring felt that this was secondary to a shocklike awareness of the patient's helplessness, whereas Jacobson believed that self-esteem could fall in a variety of ways, at times due to an as yet undefined psychosomatic factor. The onset of the disorder in these views is preceded by the subject's becoming aware of the unlikelihood of obtaining or maintaining an ideal state of well-being. Joffe and Sandler[26,27] stated that such an awareness of helplessness can be so painful and threatening that the subject fears an exhaustion of all available psychological resources in the near future and loses a sense of self-confidence. The seriously depressed subject experiences his *actual* state as so far removed from his *ideal* state of well-being that his survival is at stake. When he feels he has no way of coping with or changing the situation, further activity seems to offer little hope of bettering his plight. Since further loss is expected, any effort seems useless, and withdrawal or conservation of energy seems to be the wisest choice. This sequence results in a progressive inhibition of ego functions as exemplified in psychomotor retardation and an inability to care for oneself (wash, eat, etc.).

How does this state of affairs come about? Precipitating factors or stress factors must react upon a specific vulnerability (psychological or biological) in the subject with sufficient intensity and duration to produce various degrees of regressive change. Figure 1 attempts to outline the stages in the development of a unipolar depressive disorder. While loss may be a precipitant, any stress which compromises the individual's ability to cope or maintain his state of well-being may precipitate an episode. Predisposing or risk factors include an underlying dependency conflict and unfavorable environmental conditions which make it extremely difficult for the subject to obtain, ask for, or accept help when caught in a life crisis. The depressive patient is handicapped even in the premorbid period by impaired object relationships characterized by hostile dependency. This configuration has previously been obscured by defensive maneuvers, especially substituting overachievement for real interpersonal satisfactions. Although the predisposed individual is apparently mature and goal-oriented in his style of ego functioning, he may in fact be overly rigid in his thinking, self-blaming in his style of coping, and unable to enjoy life as an ongoing process. There is the persistence of infantile omnipotence, that is, the expectation of achieving some ideal state, which makes the acceptance of life truly impossible. The accumulation of stresses, often losses, appears to play a role in the sense that the subject is in a more vulnerable state if a second stress is applied before a prior one is adequately overcome. If the stress cannot be dealt with, the mounting of tension and psychic pain engenders feelings of worry, helplessness, and hopelessness, along with mood changes of deepening pessimism. At this point one sometimes sees the

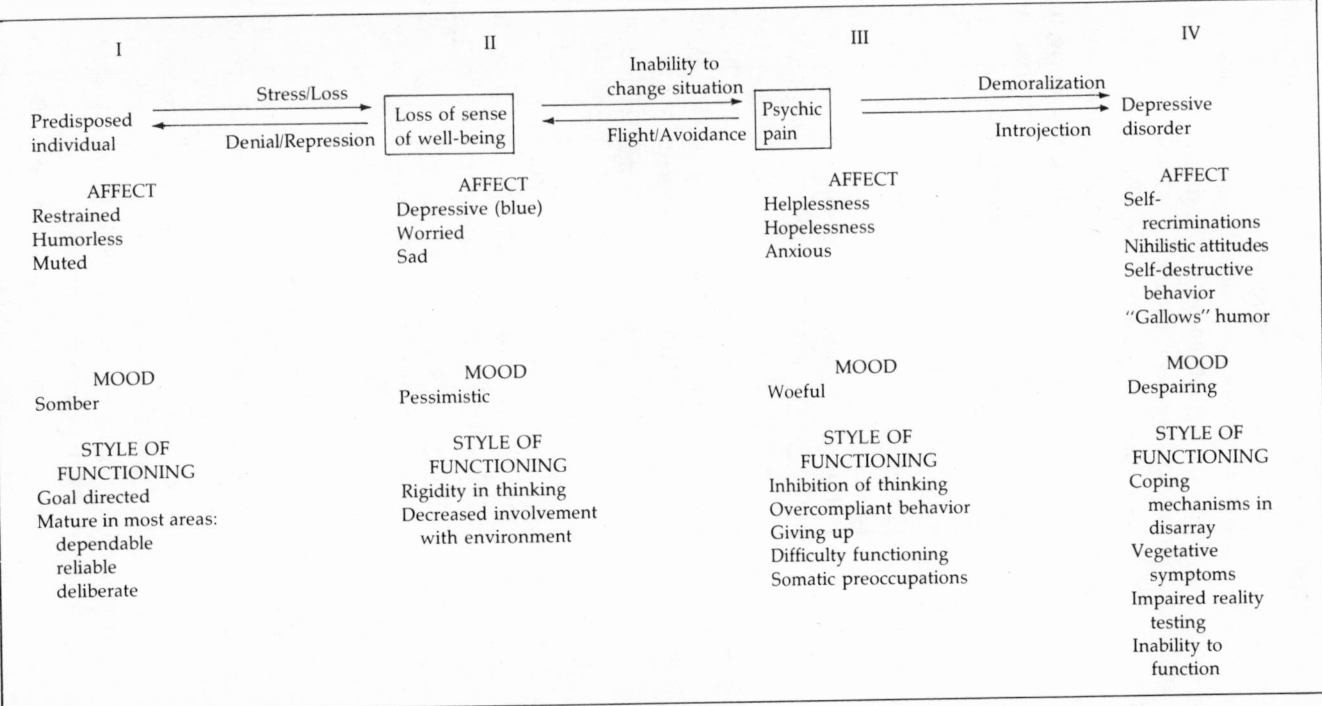

Figure 1. A schema of four stages in the development of a depressive disorder. Each shift of one stage to the right represents a regressive step or a deepening into the depressive or nodal point along this continuum. The arrows to the left indicate the operation of several coping mechanisms or defenses which have a thrust in the direction indicated. Introjection appears to be a coping mechanism which confounds the patient's equilibrium, because introjection appears to contribute to some of the most serious depressive symptomatology rather than to protect the patient, even temporarily, as does flight, avoidance, denial, and repression.

progressive unfolding of symptoms which include inhibition of thinking, hostile outbursts, social withdrawal, and, eventually, unmistakable evidence of delusions, vegetative symptoms, and suicidal preoccupation or attempts when psychic pain is unbearable.

This sequence does not occur in this form in each episode of regression in the life of every depressive patient, but it does represent a recurrent pattern for some patients with a unipolar endogenous type of depressive illness. Each episode does not develop into the full-blown clinical state we are describing. In Figure 1, we suggest that self-blame is necessary for the full development of the syndrome. By self-blame we mean directing anger against the self for being unable to respond. In our view, self-blame should be distinguished from guilt. Although there is psychic pain upon realizing that one is hopeless and helpless in maintaining one's self or self-confidence, the full depressive disorder does not necessarily follow from this realization. Rather, the depressive fails to comprehend the events surrounding him; that is, he suffers from an additional sense of demoralization. This carries with it the conviction that, whatever his previous ways of coping and adapting, he can no longer find any acceptable way of functioning or any meaning in his life. There is a regressive change in ego and superego functions. It has been generally believed that in the psychology of depression "the fault" is experienced as within the person himself. The depressive has a strong need to be "omnipotent," an omnipotence he shares with some outside "object." When he begins to fail, he attempts to rationalize his position and to assign some reason for his predicament. Since he does not know the reason or cannot accept it, he eventually concludes that it is "all his fault." His own frustrated rage is directed upon himself, which also saves the object. This process is reflected in the cognitive distortions described by Beck. The persistence of infantile omnipotence accounts for the depressive's failure to understand realistically what has happened. To preserve good, omnipotent outside sources of supply, he blames himself, maintaining an unconscious fantasy that the situation could be or should have been changed by someone. Blame in this sense replaces a search for a balanced understanding of the significant events. There must be then a sense of failure and self-blame to produce the major symptoms characteristic of the depressive syndrome, the sense of inferiority, self-recriminations, and feelings of inadequacy which are often complicated by shame and humiliation for not being able to function. The depressive even contends he caused his illness and is, therefore, to blame for it.

IMPLICATIONS FOR THERAPY

We have commented on the importance of self-recriminations and self-blame in the psychology of depressive disorders. Similarly, in therapy this becomes a danger to the treatment which can subvert supportive and exploratory efforts if its presence is not carefully noted and dealt with. The depressive's attempt at insight can be, in part, a pathological attempt to explore environmental factors and interpersonal relationships for the purpose of blaming either himself or others for his condition. In addition to requiring alertness to the management of blame, the psychotherapy of depressive disorders requires that one be alert to the problems of reassurance and dependency.

Many patients with depressive disorders are reluctant to come to psychotherapists for help. If they are willing to come for psychotherapy, they may be reluctant to take antidepressive medication. This is rationalized by the attitude that such medication will interfere with their psychotherapy. Underlying is a self-punitive impulse to punish oneself for being sick.

When a depressed patient is forced to come for help because of the intensity of his suffering, he feels forced into acknowledging more than the reality of his temporary disability. His illness confirms for him his own distorted self-appraisal that there is nothing that can be or should be done for him. Suffering from a state of despair, he believes in its inevitability and persistence. The despair that he sees objectified in his illness is a self-fulfilling prophecy. He feels responsible for it and will not see it as an end point of a pathological condition but rather the result of his own actions. In one sense he is all too willing to come for therapy for the purpose of finding the "cause" of his problem. He believes there is a cause—namely, that he is to blame for what has befallen him.

Because of these beliefs, effective reassurance is difficult to give to the depressive patient in the beginning of the treatment relationship. If the therapist states that he understands what is wrong with the patient and wishes to help him, the patient often misunderstands this offer. Given the patient's feelings of hopelessness and helplessness, the therapist must be, according to the patient's pathological views, either foolish, omnipotent, or deliberately misleading. This does not afford the therapist a good position from which to work effectively with his patient. Reassurance to the patient implies that the therapist is minimizing the problem and might not be willing to stick with the patient long enough to help him with his difficulties. The patient easily arrives at this pathological conclusion since for years he has defensively denied and minimized his emotional problems. The depressive wants to convince himself that he never had a problem in the first place.

The depressive patient often has a life history of being reliable and independent. He cannot say that he has been unable to trust in human relationships and receive support and warmth from them. He does not know, nor can he tolerate knowing, that he has turned away from people, friends, and parents throughout his life and that his successes have not brought him a sense of fulfillment. Because psychotherapeutic help involves feeling less independent and requires that the patient receive something of value from another individual, the process and nature of psychotherapy causes conflict for the depressed patient. He would like to believe in help, but he does not. Much of his nihilism and pessimism are tests to find out what the therapist believes is possible for the patient before the patient actually entrusts himself to the treatment relationship.

The problems of blame, false reassurance, and pseudoindependence are rediscovered in the treatment relationship because they reflect the lifelong disabilities of the depressive, derived from his unresolved problems of omnipotence, dependency, and inability to be responsible for his own life. These problems are discovered in the psychotherapy of the depressed patient in ways that severely test the confidence of the therapist. The therapist is confronted with the patient's helplessness, which is expressed and projected onto the therapy by the patient's questioning whether the therapist will be able to help. Then again, the patient might improve for the sake of the therapist as a transference phenomenon in the treatment situation. This initial improvement will be eventually tested and found wanting, since frustration in the therapy is inevitable when the therapist cannot produce the magic omnipotence wanted and sought by the patient. The therapist's patience and realistic attitudes are always challenged by the patient's complaints and suffering, which are unconsciously intended to provoke guilt in the therapist and wrest from the therapist a magical cure. The therapist must recognize the anger implied by these complaints and not respond to it by counteraggression. An angry response from the therapist can be extremely frightening to the patient since it threatens to disrupt the relationship and once again confirm for the patient the painfulness of close interpersonal contact.

Psychotherapy for the depressed patient requires a lengthy commitment. Its utility has been the subject of considerable research, which is in part reported in Chapter 13. Though the psychotherapeutic problems raised by treatment of depression are considerable, the value of and need for such efforts seem clear.

REFERENCES

1. Akiskal HS, McKinney WT: Overview of recent research in depression: Integration of ten conceptual models into a comprehensive clinical frame. *Arch. Gen. Psychiatry 32:*285–305, 1975.
2. Abraham K: Notes on the psychoanalytic investigation and treatment of manic-depressive insanity and allied conditions (1911). In: *Selected Papers on Psychoanalysis.* London, Hogarth Press, 1927.
3. Freud S: Mourning and melancholia. *Standard Edition,* Vol. 14, pp. 243–258. London, Hogarth Press, 1957.
4. Beck AT: *The Diagnosis and Management of Depression.* Philadelphia, University of Pennsylvania Press, 1973.
5. Fenichel O: Depression and mania. In: *The Psychoanalytic Theory of Neurosis.* New York, Norton, 1945.
6. Mendelson M: *Psychoanalytic Concepts of Depression* (2nd ed.). New York, Spectrum, 1974.
7. Abraham K: A short study of the development of the libido, viewed in the light of mental disorders. In: *Selected Papers on Psychoanalysis.* London, Hogarth Press, 1927.
8. Rado S: The problem of melancholia. *Int. J. Psychoanal. 9:*420–438, 1928.
9. Rado S: Psychodynamics of depression from the etiologic point of view. *Psychosom. Med. 13:*51–55, 1951.
10. Bibring E: The mechanism of depression. In: Greenacre P (ed): *Affective Disorders.* New York, International Universities Press, 1953.
11. Zetzel ER: The predisposition to depression. *J. Can. Psychiat. Assoc. Suppl. 11:*236–249, 1966.
12. Freud S: Inhibitions, symptoms and anxiety. *Standard Edition.* Vol. 20, pp. 77–175. London, Hogarth Press, 1959.
13. Rubinfine DL: Notes on a theory of depression. *Psychoanal. Quart. 37:*400–417, 1968.
14. Segal H: *Introduction to the Work of Melanie Klein* (2nd ed.). New York, Basic Books, 1973.
15. Klein M: Mourning and manic depressive states. *Int. J. Psychoanal. 21:*125–153, 1940.
16. Winnicott DW: The depressive position in normal emotional development. In: *Collected Papers.* London, Hogarth Press, 1958.
17. Cohen MB, Baker G, Cohen RA et al.: An intensive study of twelve cases of manic-depressive psychosis. *Psychiatry. 17:*103–138, 1954.
18. Mahler MG: Notes on the development of basic moods: The depressive affect. In: Loewenstein RM, Newman LM, Schur M, Solnit AJ (eds): *Psychoanalysis—A General Psychology.* New York, International Universities Press, 1966.
19. Jacobson E: *Depression: Comparative Studies of Normal, Neurotic and Psychotic Conditions.* New York, International Universities Press, 1971.

20. Beck AT: Thinking and depression. I. Idiosyncratic content and cognitive distortions. *Arch. Gen. Psychiatry 9:*324–333, 1963.
21. Brown GW, Harris T, Copeland JR: Depression and loss. *Br. J. Psychiatry 130:*1–18, 1977.
22. Hartmann H: The mutual influences in the development of ego and id. *Psychoanal. Study Child. 7:*9–30, 1952.
23. Feighner JP, Robins E, Guze SR et al.: Diagnostic criteria for use in psychiatric research. *Arch. Gen. Psychiatry 26:*57–63, 1972.
24. Schildkraut JJ, Klein DF: The classification and treatment of depressive disorders. In: Shader RI (ed): *Manual of Psychiatric Therapeutics.* Boston, Little, Brown, 1975.
25. Gero G: The construction of depression. *Int. J. Psychoanal. 17:*423–461, 1936.
26. Joffe WG, Sandler J: Notes on pain, depression and individuation. *Psychoanal. Study Child. 20:*394–424, 1966.
27. Joffe WG, Sandler J: Comments on the psychoanalytic psychology of adaptation, with special reference to the role of affects and the representational world. *Int. J. Psychoanal. 49:*445–454, 1968.

10

Affective Disorders in Children and Adolescents with Special Emphasis on Depression

E. JAMES ANTHONY

That fantastic great old scholar of the seventeenth century, Robert Burton (who could rightly claim to be the first psychopathologist), set it down in Part I, Section III, Subsection IV, of his *Anatomy of Melancholy*[1] that maids, virgins, nuns, barren women, and widows were especially prone to insomnia, troublesome sleep, dejection of mind, discontent, weariness, grieving, and weeping "without any manifest cause." As matters are developing today, we might very well have needed to add children to his list of vulnerable individuals or, at any rate, if we are to maintain his sex bias, little girls. He would have been a little surprised that contemporary men also frequently succumb to this "brutish kind of dotage" from the effects, presumably, of "black bile" (or its modern neurochemical equivalent). At that time, children were not supposed to suffer from anything but mental deficiency, and it is only in the past century that they were deemed capable of developing psychopathology and only in the last couple of decades that they were judged to be depressed. It seems that as adults became more aware of children as individuals, they also became aware of the wide range of affective disorders that they could manifest. A worldwide interest has developed in childhood depression with three points of view predominating: that it did not exist except in the minds of certain overly sensitive clinicians who detected such affects in almost every patient; that it existed in different forms throughout childhood; and, finally, that it was a plausible hypothesis to be tested open-mindedly. Before one tested this

E. JAMES ANTHONY • Division of Child Psychiatry, Washington University School of Medicine, St. Louis, Missouri.

hypothesis, it seemed important to define and limit the concept and thus not render it too inclusive. The need to look for it is critical to the prospect of finding it. Malmquist[2] reported that, although child patients may both look and behave in a depressed way, the diagnosis of depression is rarely entertained. One reason for this is that the diagnosis has often been omitted from standard psychiatric classifications. Thus, Malmquist has, himself, proposed a detailed classification for childhood depressions.

If it does exist, and I for one believe it does, it is certainly not as a unitary phenomenon but as a syndrome or constellation of symptoms that have come together in a logical pattern. If it does exist as such, it should relate, on the one hand, to the normal range of affective expression in the child and, on the other, to the clinical disturbances of affect appearing later in the adult. These two continuities could be reasonable to expect although they are still far from proven. A third continuity could be with the affective disturbances found in the universe of children through epidemiological inquiry, and a fourth continuity could be between the anxiety and depressive disorders.

In the current work on childhood depression, its existence has been taken for granted and three models have been used to investigate it more fully. The empirical model runs along medical lines and has attempted to examine antecedent conditions, concomitant disturbances, natural course, typologies, and therapeutic response, more especially to drugs. The adult model of depression has exerted a powerful and binding influence on the work of the empiricist. In general, he has attempted to take the knowns of the adult condition and to extrapolate from them what might be expected in the child. Hidden in this approach is the view of the child as essentially a miniature adult whose responses, in the main, will resemble the adult response somewhat miniaturized. Out of this has grown a number of scales derived from grown-up sources that have tried to give us an objectively reliable and valid measure of depression in children. External ratings, focusing on behavioral aspects of the affective response, have not furnished satisfactory inter-rater reliabilities (I am thinking here of Rutter's Scale used in his Isle-of-Wight studies), and inquiries carried out following the administration of self-rating scales have often left the uneasy feeling that the children have not comprehended what is being asked. Moreover, such scales are often validated against the clinical judgment which Connors[3] has described as the correlation of the mysterious with the unknown.

Other empirical attempts to define and to limit the diagnosis of affective disorder are still on the drawing board awaiting a reliable instrument. They include the follow-up of affectively disturbed children into adult life, prevalence studies of the affective disturbances in the families of children with affective disturbances (presumably to tap the degree of genetic loading), and epidemiological surveys employing adequate representative samples. The supposition in all this is that affective disorders do exist in children and simply need to be ascertained and assessed.

Therapeutic tests suffer from the same drawbacks of diagnosis and the assumption of a unitary disease entity: depressed children are those who respond to antidepressant medication overlooking the fact that drug administration involves the setting up of complex response systems within the body and mind of the recipient. Furthermore, children often give paradoxical and unexpected responses to drugs: thus, they may respond to stimulant drugs with absence of euphoria and to antidepressant drugs with an absence of mood change (although an accompanying enuresis may improve). They do not show a depressive response to corticosteroids. Major and quite unwarranted conclusions may sometimes be drawn from the drug effects. The group of enuretics that clear up are then referred to as depressed enuretics and enuresis then becomes a prime example of masked depression so that masked depression rapidly becomes a fact when it is still an interesting hypothesis.

The focus on externals is to some extent justifiable since children seem rapidly to convert affect into activity, acting out, and somatic dysfunction. But, in remembering this, it is also important to bear in mind that a host of internal events are also occurring at the same time and may be at variance with outer manifestations.

This, however, leads us to consider another model that has been used to explore childhood depression—a psychodynamic one in which internal conflict plays an important role. This model, in the strong tradition of psychoanalysis, attempts to relate the first few years of childhood to what develops in the subsequent phases of the life cycle. The classical Abraham–Freud theory stemmed from the analysis of melancholic patients where psychotic regression was a prominent feature. It was largely based on a superego pathology and incorporated such concepts as aggression turned against the self, excessive orality, narcissistic injury, marked ambivalence, masochism, and the internalization of a lost object. Dispositional factors were thought to be constitutional excesses of narcissism and orality. For structural reasons, in that the child's mental apparatus lacks the mature elaborations found in the adult, psychoanalysts have concluded either that children can not become melancholic (and this is certainly true in its psychotic sense) or that the theory cannot fit the picture of childhood depression. A later theory, formulated by Bibring,[4] is based on a psychology of the ego involving the regulation of self-esteem. It is much easier for the child clinician to understand his particular case of depression in the context of this framework.

With the dynamic model, there is less emphasis on differentiating clearly between normal and abnormal depression (viewed on a continuum), between endogenous and exogenous (since all depressions would be regarded as originating in reactions to loss, injury, disappointment, or hurt), between primary and secondary (meaning secondary to some other physical or mental disorder), or between neurotic and psychotic (since melancholia is outside the range of childhood disorders).

The internal workings of a depression may be disclosed through fantasies, drawings, projections, dreams, and the suicidal ideation that is found in about 20% of latency children manifesting other evidence of depression. All these subjective deductions tend to have a similar content that is again understandable in the light of Bibring's theory: the characters in the various themes all tend to feel injured, frustrated, trapped, empty, and catastrophically helpless. Anxiety cases differ in that the various situations are still threatening rather than occurring. Their presence in a masked depression is presently taken as proof of the depressive nature of the disorder.

For those actually working with children and adolescents, the developmental model becomes something in the nature of a categorical imperative. Clinicians working with such patients are well aware of the continuous changes and modifications occurring over time not only with regard to normal but also abnormal conditions. The child at different stages presents himself with different clinical faces involving different constellations of symptoms. This is very true of the affective syndromes. One would expect, therefore, that clinical depression would manifest itself in a variety of ways through childhood and adolescence. The developmental psychologist is also acutely conscious of the child's "developmental environment," meaning by this the changing input from parents, families, and culture. Parents may suffer from affective disturbances and feed their affects and concomitant erratic behavior into the developmental environment and these may influence the child differently at different stages of his development. Chronically depressed mothers may be as unavailable to the child emotionally as rejecting mothers. It is through the parents that children are taught or learn how to manifest illness and it is from them that they pick up gradually an appropriate language to represent as accurately as possible their complaints. Families, like cultures, may facilitate or impede the expression of affects. In what I have called "open" families, affects are permitted free rein so that a child can mourn or grieve or express his disappointments with freedom and with encouragement. This is often in singular contrast with "closed" families where aggression is poorly handled and mostly disguised, where sexual matters are taboo, where references to death are considered alarming, and where children may be a little unhappy but never depressed. If they are depressed, they learn quickly not to show it.

The clinical picture of the affective disorders is also influenced by the cognitive level so that the child's competence and coping skills and problem-solving capacities help to shape the clinical picture.[5] A number of important factors are subsumed under this general category. As the child develops, there are changes in his ability to introspect, to communicate his feelings, to make meaningful causal connections, to place his subjective experiences in a time perspective, and to generate operational concepts of illness. At an earlier stage, his feelings, like his thoughts, tend to be syncretic and amorphous. It is only as he differentiates within himself and develops a sense of self and identity that he can begin to resemble the adult depressive.

Three sets of data are of importance in buttressing the developmental model: retrospective studies of the childhood of adult depressed patients, follow-up studies of child depressed patients, and studies of children at high risk for affective disorders. Such children can be identified in two ways: first, they may be children of manic-depressive parents (a study in which I am currently engaged), or, second, they may be recognized as predisposed to affective disorder because of certain antecedents in their history. In children with a high genetic risk, two separate groups may be identified: those with lithium-responding parents who developed manic-depression early and whose family history is strong in manic-depression; and those children with parents who developed manic-depression late and have a negative family history and only a minimal response to lithium. In my investigation, we are now experiencing adolescent breakdowns, predominantly of a depressive nature, in children of the first category, starting in early puberty, as in the case of Virginia Woolf, who described her adolescent attacks as "breakdowns in miniature."[6] We have also observed episodic depressions in children of the second category but these seem more in the nature of environmental transmission since they often coincide with severe depressions in the parent. (These would be similar to a *folie a deux.)*[5] In the six breakdowns in our sample so far, suicidal attempts have played a prominent part.

The clinical recognition of children at high risk for affective disorder involves a complicated set of dispositional criteria.

DISPOSITIONAL FACTORS

Psychoanalytic theory has recently placed less stress on such allegedly "constitutional" predispositions as orality and has focused its attention more on intrapsychic developments in the first five years of life. Klein[7] has postulated the normal occurrence of a "depressive position" in the first year of life, associated with a manic defense, that, when unresolved, sets up a depressive tendency that can culminate eventually in a depressive psychosis. Benedek[8] has put forward an elaborate transactional theory involving three generations, grandmother, mother, and infant, in which an intense conflict of ambivalence leads to the formation of a "depressive constellation" that predisposes to a variety of affective disorders. Mahler[9] has described the emergence of a basic depressive mood in certain children during the third subphase of rapprochement with mothers who basically reject the toddler. This basic mood consists of moodiness, neediness, demandingness, clingingness, loneliness, feelings of unwantedness, and a tendency to respond to frustration with helplessness and hopelessness. The same depressive tendency would arise, according to Engel,[10] when there is any disturbance of the core mechanism of conversation–withdrawal leading to an exaggerated inhibitory and withdrawal tendency. Two other theorists, Spitz[11] and Bowlby,[12] believe that the *actual* experience of loss can set up anaclitic and bereavement reactions that bring about withdrawal, despair, and detachment. They do not say to what extent this early experience sensitizes the child and adolescent and renders him prone to depressive responses. Jacobson[13] has resurrected the Abraham's theory of "primal disappointment" occurring during the oedipal period to account for a depressive tendency. It should be noticed that the term *depression* is used fairly loosely in all these suggestions. None of these would approximate to the depressions occurring later. By using the word to describe a negative or withdrawal reaction one tends to prejudge the issue of whether the early and late sets of reactions are in continuity.

In addition to these intrapsychic dispositional factors, there are more objective ones that have been cited in the literature: a family history of affective disorder, a history of repeated or protracted separations, rejecting and disparaging parents, the experience of loss especially with limited opportunities for mourning, the occurrence of minor mood disorders such as boredom, nostalgia, and moodiness, and the manifest need for immediate surrogation in the face of transient separations. A dispositional test has been reported in which 10% to 15% of children (roughly the number felt to be depression-prone) respond to stimulant drugs (amphetamine) with weepiness, sadness, withdrawal, and an adult depressive appearance accompanied by self-recriminations that Connors[3] has referred to as the appearance of "instant superego."

CORE FACTORS IN THE GENESIS OF AFFECTIVE DISORDERS IN CHILDREN AND ADOLESCENTS

Depressive listings of innumerable symptoms often tell us very little except that the depressive affect like the anxiety affect can invade and pervade with a large variety of mental and physical disorders. In so-called "masked" depression or depressive equivalent, the depressive affect has supposedly reached an abnormal level and is then confronted by a series of defense and compensatory mechanisms—obsessional devices, manic reactions, somatic disturbances—that vary with the stage of development. In the earlier stages, there are dysfunctions of eating and sleeping (infantile disturbances of the sleep rhythm have been included by some among dispositional indices); in the middle years, learning disturbances and school phobias may be present; and in adolescence, acting out the delinquency may occur.[14] Critics have felt that almost every known symptom in child psychiatry has been linked directly or indirectly to depression (and the same of course is true of anxiety). Factor analyses of symptom lists do little more than confirm and reinforce biased preconceptions.

The affective disturbance can be best understood, in my view, in terms of imbalances in a number of basic regulatory mechanisms that include the following:

1. The regulation of self-esteem (between superiority and inferiority).
2. The regulation of hedonic capacity (between pleasure and unpleasure).
3. The regulation of self-confidence (between omnipotence and helplessness).
4. The regulation of hopefulness (between optimism and pessimism).
5. The regulation of psychic input and output (between fullness and emptiness).
6. The overall regulation of affect (between elation and depression, between euphoria and dysphoria).

These regulations presuppose a biological core determined by hormonal and autonomic mechanisms surrounded by psychobiological factors associated with conservation–withdrawal, with overlayers of psychological responses of ego and self to the more nuclear events.

PRECOCIOUS ADULT AFFECTIVE PSYCHOSES IN CHILDHOOD

No well-authenticated case of depressive psychosis as seen in the adult has been reported in children. Anthony and Scott[15] reviewed the literature on manic-depressive psychosis in childhood and came to the conclusion that it was extremely rare and that their own case represented an anomaly. However, when loosely defined, diagnosis of manic-depression has been made with surprising frequency. What this often referred to was a cycloid tendency that might or might not be an antecedent to the adult psychosis. Sometimes the amplifications or "cycloid deviations" represented embryonic forms of the later illness. One of the precursors described was a delirious manic or depressive outburst occurring during pyrexial illness in the child. Making use of ten criteria, only four cases met the standard. The criteria included a family history of manic-depression, a cyclothymic tendency, periodic occurrences of micropsychoses, an extroverted type of personality, and a lack of correlation between affective disturbance and environmental events. Also included was an absence of organic pathology.

ADOLESCENT DEPRESSION

Less debatable forms of depression begin in adolescence—one depression has been referred to by some psychodynamic theorists as a stage of mourning which is gradually worked through during the course of adolescence and is related to the loss of childhood and the final renunciation of parental objects. At this time, one may see early cases of manic-depression, depressive "breakdowns in miniature" in cases of high genetic risk for manic-depression, typical adolescent depressions associated with separation–individuation and identity problems having their origin in preoedipal life, normal depressive moodiness characteristic of this stage, and schizoaffective disorders beginning with a depressive coloring.

Anthony[16] has described two typical syndromes of adolescent depression, the one seemingly having its roots in the first three years of life and the other characteristically beginning with a depressive turmoil during middle latency. The first is based on a heavily symbiotic relationship with an omnipotent, sadistic mother. These patients are extremely dependent and demonstrate considerable lowered self-esteem, shame, and feelings of weakness. The second type is characterized by a punitive superego and guilt. Anger toward parents for not fulfilling their idolized images is directed against the self resulting in self-disgust and possibly self-destructive behavior. The psychoanalytic treatment of such depressions, without the use of drugs, involves a great deal of patience, persistence, and forbearance on the part of the therapist, who is likely at times to experience minor depressions himself during the course of the treatment.

The suicide rate escalates alarmingly toward midadolescence together with the use of drugs, which has sometimes been equated with self-medication for the increasing experience of depression. Many individuals today are struggling through adolescence with the help of antidepressants and stimulants used to gross excess but sometimes titrated in relation to the mood disturbance. Vulnerable adolescents, that is, those with a marked dispositional tendency, tend to show at this time an increase in suicidal ideation and depressive fantasy prior to any depressive "breakdown."

MANIFEST AND LATENT DEPRESSIONS DURING CHILDHOOD AND ADOLESCENCE

Given the depressive predisposition, the depressive disorder may manifest itself off and on during various critical times within the first two decades of life. For long periods, the depression may remain subterranean until certain specific environmental precipitants evoke its reappearance. Two clinical examples will suffice to illustrate what happens.

CASE 1. This was the case of a difficult baby who became a difficult toddler and then a difficult child to whom no one could put a diagnosis, except to say that he was a problem child who seemed to generate his own difficulties and went through his early development trailing clouds of diverse symptoms. He seemed chronically discontented and dissatisfied with himself and his lot and found it difficult to make or retain friends since he soon withdrew from them. He began psychotherapy at the age of nine and made little or no contact with his therapist, sitting mostly silent with his head bowed down. About a year later, he came to his session one day and said: "I keep having a dream ever since I was little and it bothers me." The therapist was inwardly delighted although he managed to look merely attentive. He had almost given up hope on this child and had begun to find the sessions terribly tedious. He had not expected much in the first place. The boy was the love child of a woman who had been deserted while she was pregnant. She had brought him up by herself for years and then she remarried and had six more children. For five years he had lived alone with his mother, having her all to himself, and now he was suddenly introduced into a complete family. This is what he told his therapist: "In the dream I have money, lots of money, but then I lose it all. Well, I don't lose it but I give it to my mother for her to keep for me and then, when I ask her back for it because I want to buy something for myself, she tells me that she has already given it to my brothers and sisters and that they have spent it and, when I complained to my parents, they said that there was nothing they could do about it. I keep having this dream over and over again." Telling the dream to the therapist released his pent-up feelings and he began to cry and then his depression for the first time became obvious. Before that no one had mentioned it because he had been so overactive but, on looking back, it was clear that he had been struggling with a latent depression most of the time. The dream was a summarizing dream in that it brought together his sense of loss and impoverishment, his sibling jealousy, and his feelings of hopelessness and helplessness. In communicating this to the therapist, he was enabling something to be done about his very human predicament.

CASE 2. This was a little boy who was very angry inside but who never let it out. His inhibition made it difficult for him to make friends. At times he looked depressed but mostly his affect was flat. He was started in psychotherapy at the age of seven and when he was eight he told his therapist that he was constantly afraid that his father might die. He even began to have dreams about his father's dying. Following this, he again became uncooperative and withdrawn and unable to use help. About a year later, quite suddenly, his father suddenly died. His tongue and his feelings were suddenly loosened and he began to talk in a very emotional way. In the session, he said to his therapist, at first without feeling and then with increasing feeling: "My father died suddenly with a heart attack five days ago. It started with chest pain." At this point he looked very miserable and began to talk about school work and the difficulties he was having learning new words. The sadness was growing and he was soon crying and sobbing. The therapist was sympathetic and supportive. He went back to school but very soon they had to expel him because his behavior had deteriorated so badly. At the session following his expulsion, he said: "I can't find any images of my father in my mind. He's so far away from me now. I am sad. I feel empty." The next session he came in looking grubby with dirty hands and clothes and remarked: "This is how I used to be. I am sad all the time." The therapist said, "I know how sad you have been since your father died," but the boy immediately interrupted him and said: "No, no, no. I was sad long before he died. I was sad all the time. I really don't know how I first came out sad." The therapist asked when he thought that he had become sad and he said, "I think I was sad when I was about two years old, but you know why? I think it was when my sister was born." In the next session, he was silent, deeply depressed, slowed down in his mental activity, and quite unable to cope with even simple everyday tasks. His condition rapidly worsened and he was admitted to the hospital.

Here we have two cases where one can almost reconstruct the whole course of depression during latent and manifest phases. In the second case, the boy was almost able to face the natural course of his disorder and to see behind the recent bereavement to the earlier depression, which stemmed from his intense feeling of losing his mother at the birth of his sister. His oedipal rivalry with his father, as reflected in his fear that his father might die, had ended in an actual oedipal triumph with the death of his father and this was too much for him to tolerate, especially since he had felt bereaved ever since the birth of his sister.

I can see why many clinicians are so convinced that affective disorders do occur in children even though they might find it difficult to demonstrate its existence to an objective investigator. They will have less difficulty in sharing their conviction about adolescent affective disorders since these are beginning to look very much like the depressions described in the textbooks, although still somewhat fluctuating and irregular in their course. In summing up, therefore, one can only reiterate that affective disorders do exist in children and adolescents; that they can exist in any child or adolescent, but that they are more likely to occur in children who are predisposed and in children at high risk for affective disorders. They are also more likely to occur in children from particular families and from particular cultures. About the biological basis for this proclivity, there is still as yet no answer, but the search has begun.

REFERENCES

1. Burton R: *The Anatomy of Melancholy.* New York, Farrar and Rinehart, 1927.
2. Malmquist C: Depressions in Childhood and Adolescence. Part I. *New Engl. J. Med. 284:*887–893, 1971.
3. Conners CK: Discussion. In: Schutterbrandt J, Raskin A (eds) *Depression in Childhood: Diagnosis, Treatment, and Conceptual Models.* New York, Raven Press, 1977.
4. Bibring E: The mechanism of depression. In: Greenacre P (ed) *Affective Disorders.* New York, International Universities Press, 1953.
5. Anthony EJ: Influence of a manic-depressive environment on the child. In: Anthony EJ, Benedek T (eds) *Depression and Human Existence.* Boston, Little, Brown, 1975.
6. Bell Q: *Virginia Woolf.* New York, Harcourt, Brace, 1972.
7. Klein M: A contribution to the psychogenesis of manic-depressive states. In: *Contributions to Psycho-Analysis.* London, Hogarth Press, 1948.
8. Benedek T: Toward the biology of the depressive constellation. *J. Am. Psychoanal. Assoc. 4:*389–427, 1956.
9. Mahler M: Notes on the development of basic moods: The depressive affect in psychoanalysis. In: Loewenstein R (ed) *Psychoanalysis—A General Psychology.* New York, International Universities Press, 1966.
10. Engel GL: Anxiety and depression-withdrawal: The primary affects of unpleasure. *Int. J. Psychoanal. 43:*89–97, 1962.
11. Spitz RA, Wolf KM: Anaclitic depression. *Psychoanal. Study Child. 2:*313–341, 1946.
12. Bowlby J: Some pathological processes set in train by early mother-child separation. *J. Ment. Sci. 99:*265–272, 1953.
13. Jacobson E: The Oedipus conflict in the development of depressive mechanisms. *Psychoanal. Q. 12:*541–560, 1943.
14. Anthony EJ: On the genesis of childhood depression. In: Anthony EJ, Gilpin D (eds) *Three Clinical Faces of Childhood.* New York, Spectrum Publications, 1976.
15. Anthony EJ, Scott P: Manic-depressive psychosis in childhood. *Child Psychology and Psychiatry. 1:*53–72, 1960.
16. Anthony EJ: Two contrasting types of adolescent depression and their treatment. *J. Am. Psychoanal. Assoc. 18:*841–859, 1970.

11

Brief Psychotherapy of Depression

PIETRO CASTELNUOVO-TEDESCO

Most individual psychotherapy falls under the rubric of brief or short-term treatment and this chapter will address its application in depression. Together with anxiety, depression is one of the fundamental human reactions of conflict and distress, so much so that in ordinary parlance unhappiness and depression are practically synonymous. With its broad range of gradations and its variety of manifestations depression is perhaps the most common of psychiatric conditions. It is seen with great frequency, not only by the psychiatrist but also, of course, by the general physician or for that matter by anyone who has occasion to deal professionally with emotionally upset persons.

Another interesting facet of depression is how it highlights the psychotherapeutic task. When we deal with depressed patients, it regularly becomes apparent that their illness has meaning within a human context. In depression perhaps even more than in other psychiatric states one is impressed with the fact that, to help the patient recover, one has to help him to unburden himself of the meaning that he attaches to his circumstances—external and internal—and to restructure this meaning into something more positive and hopeful. In depression one becomes particularly aware that patients have *plaints* as well as complaints, that they have *grievances* as well as griefs, and that one must provide an airing and hopefully find some resolution for these plaints and grievances to help the patient to feel better. Depressed patients typically feel that life has used them ill and has deprived them of their full share. How do we go about helping these patients achieve a more positive and hopeful view of themselves and their circumstances? The chapter will attempt to address this issue.

PIETRO CASTELNUOVO-TEDESCO • Department of Psychiatry, Vanderbilt University School of Medicine, Nashville, Tennessee.

First, a brief but necessary digression: What do we mean by *brief treatment* and for what depressive conditions is it suitable?

Brief treatment is a flexible concept and not everyone agrees exactly as to what it covers. The time dimension alone is not very satisfactory to describe this form of treatment, but I am using the term here to refer to something less than 25 psychotherapeutic interviews, i.e., lasting in most cases somewhere between 3 and 6 months.[1] Sometimes less than 10 sessions are needed: for example, 3, 4, or 5 would suffice. The usual frequency of visits is once or twice per week, but occasionally more frequent visits are necessary, if the symptoms are particularly acute. I will come back to this later.

For what conditions is brief treatment suitable? Perhaps it is easiest if we mention first those that should be considered unsuitable. Here I am referring specifically to psychotic depressions, i.e., those that are very severe, and to those neurotic depressions that are chronic and where the personality as a whole is deeply involved in the need to suffer. Patients who are outspokenly self-centered or passive–dependent, masochistic, or self-destructive generally are not good prospects for brief treatment. Treatment for these patients tends to be prolonged and it is generally inappropriate to think of short-term measures. Which patients, then, are left as suitable for brief treatment? We could list primarily the milder neurotic reactions, some of the more complicated grief reactions that are slow to resolve spontaneously, and the situational reactions that are characterized mainly by depression. How do we determine patients' suitability? The principal yardstick is a simple one to apply. We consider whether the patient, despite his discomfort from depressive symptomatology, remains capable of functioning in his accustomed social role. In other words, we assess his effectiveness and observe whether psychologically he is still on his feet, so to speak, and not supine. This is a most important criterion for selecting patients appropriately for brief treatment, one that cannot be overemphasized. The patient can still work, earn a living, run a house, or do whatever he or she usually does. He is capable of friendship and has maintained functioning relationships with other people, even though these may be unsatisfactory or conflictual in certain respects. Also the situational aspects of the difficulty are well in evidence in that the patient himself usually recognizes that the symptoms have arisen in response to some emotionally upsetting event or events.

This must be qualified by saying that, even when the patient is aware in a general way that his trouble is related to certain upsetting events that have just occurred, he does not really understand their meaning and there are crucial aspects of the difficulty which he consistently avoids. It is important to differentiate between the patient's having *knowledge* of the precipitants (which he often does) and being able to appreciate the *significance* that these events have for him (which usually he does not, or at most he does in a very limited way). In the milder cases this often includes even a lack of awareness by the patient that his difficulties in fact constitute a depression. The patient's ability to appreciate the meaning of his circumstances is intimately tied to his capacity to feel and express the relevant emotions. Improvement specifically takes place as meanings are clarified and as painful emotions are discharged and understood in the context of the therapeutic relationship. As an example of the need to acquaint the patient with the meaning of his difficulties, let me mention a case that I had occasion to see not long ago. An attractive and youthful woman of 40 was referred by her internist because of "loss of libido." This bit of medical jargon was the internist's way of describing that she had come to dislike sex and was avoiding sexual relations with her husband as much as possible. She was concerned and puzzled by her change in attitude because in earlier years her sexual relations with him had been active, frequent, and pleasurable. The basic story, once it emerged, proved quite simple. Some years back, because of a recurrent manic-depressive disorder, the patient's husband had stopped working and the patient had had to go to work to support the family. Despite her best efforts, money had been tight. The patient had resented going to work and being deprived of the economic standing that she would have enjoyed by now if her husband had been able to pursue his occupation. She also reported with some bitterness that, while her husband considered himself unable to work and failed even to help at home with chores, at night his interest in sex and his energy were undiminished. Her resentment of the situation was such that she no longer felt able to participate in lovemaking. She felt completely turned off. The important point of this story is that none of this was conscious to her. She thought she had developed some kind of strange and to her unexplained sexual difficulty. She was not aware that she was suffering from a depression and that her problem centered on her profound disappointment in her husband and her marriage.

I want to stress that the depressed patient needs not only an opportunity to grieve but also to understand, i.e., he needs to obtain some grasp of what it is that he is grieving about, to discover what he thinks he has lost. In other words, it is not enough to give the patient a chance to express himself fully and freely (even though this is essential). He also needs to be told, i.e., to have explained in an appropriate and sympathetic way what he is missing and what his loss contains. This should be done as early as possible, i.e., as soon as some measure of understanding is available to be communicated to the patient. Otherwise, the patient may find himself talking on and on and getting nothing back from a physician who sits passively and silently listening to a long tale of woe. The result frequently is increasing discouragement, deepening depression, and a mounting sense of alienation from the therapist, who is felt (perhaps correctly) to be out of touch with the situation.

Here I will not go into a detailed description of the depressive symptomatology. This has already been discussed in earlier chapters. However, I would like to emphasize again how varied a group this is and how much ordinarily is included under the term *depression.* Freud[2] distinguished the patients who are grieving and feel sad from those who are dejected and have lost their self-esteem. There are also patients who complain primarily of apathy, a sense of emptiness and futility, a feeling of being out of touch with things and people. While these are often described as depressed, many are really schizoid persons. In other words, they are detached and have shallow affects. There is also a large group of patients whose depression manifests itself mainly through somatic equivalents. These patients are usually seen first by the internist rather than by the psychiatrist. My impression is that brief treatment is noticeably *in*effective when one is dealing with a basically schizoid illness. The other categories of patients tend to do well if one adheres to the criteria of selection that I have mentioned, namely continued capacity for social functioning, presence of fairly clear-cut precipitating circumstances, and a depression of only moderate severity, fairly recent onset, and without deep-seated characterologic features (specifically, patients who do not show strong masochistic traits and a chronic need to suffer).

In order to talk meaningfully about treatment, we need a framework for understanding these depressive reactions. As a general model it is useful to keep in mind that they occur in response to the loss of something that has special value for the patient, that is close to his heart. This "something" may be a loved person, a job, social status or approval, or some long-cherished hopes. The loss need not have occurred in reality; in some cases it may be simply a threatened loss or even a phantasied one. The question of loss inevitably involves the problem of *disappointment,* which is crucial for the depressed patient, and disappointment inevitably involves the issue of *regret,* i.e., that of missed opportunities and what might have been done or should have been done (both by the patient and by others who were close to him). Let me stress the significance of both disappointment and regret. The word *disappointment* is extremely helpful in our own private thinking about depression. It clarifies matters if we establish for ourselves that a depressed man is first and foremost a *disappointed* man. But, in addition, the word *disappointment* is a useful one to employ in talking with the patient because it easily leads into a discussion of the frustrations he has experienced, the longings and expectations that have gone unfulfilled, and the anger that he has felt toward important persons who—in his eyes at least—have failed him. Thus there are vengeful thoughts directed at those whom the patient holds responsible for his difficulties. The presence of these bitter thoughts may not be readily apparent because often they are only fleetingly conscious and are submerged in layers of guilt.

Please note the following: someone who is depressed feels that he has been let down or that he has let himself down. Speaking with the patient about his feelings of regret helps him not only to express the reproaches that he has toward himself and toward others but also leads to a clearer understanding of his values and expectations. Ultimately it leads to a reassessment of his situation and what he can still do to salvage it. Taking responsive action is better than suffering passively. The ability to take some action, even if it has limited results, is therapeutic and is associated usually with clinical improvement, yet taking action is difficult for the depressed patient, who is inclined rather to submit to his misery and bemoan his fate. Often one notes that the patient has difficulty not only taking action but also considering any alternative ways of coping with his predicament. The depressed patient typically feels immobilized or presents his situation as if it had no solution. Ahead of him is a large sign that reads, "No exit," but, as the patient begins to give consideration to alternatives, this tends to dilute the atmosphere of hopelessness with which he has surrounded himself.

In addition to the generalization about the depressed man as a disappointed man, I want to discuss three other generalizations that commonly are encountered in everyday thinking about depression.

First is the one about the depressed man as an *angry* man. Depressed people certainly tend to be angry people, yet therapeutically it is not very helpful to consider the anger by itself, as something unitary and basic in the patient's makeup. Therapists who operate in terms of this conceptual model often are busily at work "releasing the patient's anger" without really appreciating that the anger itself is a reaction to the disappointments and the hurts the patient has experienced and which still underlie the anger. In its crudest form, a therapeutic approach of this sort often means advice to the patient that what he needs to do is to blow off steam, let himself go, or tell his wife, his boss, or whomever might be involved precisely how he feels. At best this results in no improvement; at worst it can have disastrous consequences. It is only when the hurts and the disappointments are acknowledged, recognized, and then realistically evaluated that the resentment can begin to be expressed in a meaningful way (primarily in the treatment setting) and finally be dissipated. If, in one's comments to the patient one stresses the anger he feels rather than the hurts and disappointments which underlie it, the patient often simply understands that he is being told he is *bad* since anger commonly is considered a reprehensible emotion. The result not infrequently is that the patient, instead of improving, becomes even more depressed.

Another important generalization about depression is the one about the depressed man as a *guilty* man. Rather than disappointed, hungering, or angry, he feels bad, wretched, and unworthy. He lacks self-esteem because he has lost the approval and support of his conscience. His disappointment—on the surface at least—is with himself, but beyond this again it is with others who, during the crisis, did not act in a way to help him maintain a good image of himself.

Of course, many gradations occur and these generalizations are not to be construed as representing pure types. In practice many blendings are seen, although we also must recognize that some patients present themselves primarily because they are disappointed, others primarily because they are angry, and still others primarily because they are guilty and ashamed. Not infrequently an important source of guilt is the resentment the patient feels toward a close person whom, on the contrary, he feels he should love (or whom he also does love). The guilt (whatever its origin) tends to attach itself to particular current events, and then it becomes very useful to air and discuss these. One must also not forget to mention a very common situation where guilt plays a significant role. I am referring to the so-called *guilty secret,* from which many patients suffer and yet which they often are very loath to divulge. In fact, frequently the doctor does not find out about the secret unless he is particularly attuned to this issue and makes special efforts to help the patient to reveal it. When we speak of a guilty secret we are not referring to something unconscious and deeply repressed but rather to something which is quite conscious or at least very near consciousness. Frequently it has to do with some kind of sexual event of which the patient feels particularly ashamed and which he has tried hard to bury in the back of his mind: for example, an illegitimate pregnancy, an extramarital affair, or a homosexual escapade. The patient tries hard to erase the memory, but often, despite his best efforts, it will not disappear and continues to have a steady, corrosive effect. The patient, if he is lucky, eventually manages to find in the physician a friend to whom he can finally unburden himself. Under optimal circumstances, the patient's confession is highly dramatic and becomes the focal point of the whole interview. At this point the patient often becomes upset and agitated as he tells the story of what he considers his misdeed. There is generally much pressure of feeling, and the patient's account tends to be interspersed with painful sobbings and statements of contrition. It is important that the patient tell in great detail the story which previously he had held back and tried to hide and that the doctor do what he can to facilitate a full discharge of feeling.

Frequently, after the dam has burst and the outpouring has begun, all one needs to do is to make sure one does not interrupt the patient until he has had his say, fully and completely. It is also important not to probe the confession prematurely for its deeper dynamic implications. It seems better to accept it quietly, with compassion, and to convey to the patient a sympathetic appreciation of his predicament. Later one reviews with him the content of his disclosures to help place the matter in a broader perspective with the goal of alleviating his guilt and stimulating constructive action. The patient's response is often impressive. Generally he experiences an almost immediate sense of relief, and many things which previously had been unclear rapidly come into focus. If the confession occurs not immediately at the beginning of treatment but some time later, one notices that the tempo of treatment becomes accelerated so that often it can be brought to an early and satisfactory conclusion. At the same time we should be aware that rapid penetration into areas which are heavily laden with guilt involves certain risks and may have undesirable effects. The patient, instead of feeling better as a result of having unburdened himself and found some measure of acceptance, may come to feel much worse, more guilty, and more depressed. This is particularly likely to occur if the patient has special problems of mistrust and tends to be suspicious of the motives of others. In these instances, the patient may well emerge from the interview feeling exposed and prematurely stripped of his defenses and may view the doctor as a persecutor who now "has the goods" on him rather than as a helping person. In other words, guilt and guilty secrets need to be handled delicately.

One final generalization concerning depression, which should not be left out, is the one about the depressed patient *as a dependent and helpless person*. These patients lack a sense of self-sufficiency, and what they lose is always the same thing, even though it takes many guises, namely, the confidence that they can pull through on their own or that those about them are willing to give them the help they feel they need so badly and which, incidentally, they regard as their due. Doubt, uncertainty, and, beyond these, mistrust are always prominent in their makeup. To some extent these issues are true for all depressed patients. However, when they are particularly outspoken and have become an important and stable part of the personality structure, the patient generally is not a good candidate for brief treatment, and other approaches requiring more time and capable of dealing with long-standing personality distortions are to be preferred.

In the brief treatment of these depressive reactions, it is important to recognize early the major characterological defenses and, *in the main,* to respect them, to leave them alone, and not to become involved in premature attempts at character analysis which are not in keeping with the circumscribed goals of brief treatment. One of the common technical errors in brief treatment is the attempt to combine symptom-relief, which is the primary goal, with haphazard thrusts at personality reconstruction. This may derive from a euphoric notion that if the doctor tinkers with basic defenses it means he is practicing analytic treatment and is offering something more sophisticated than workaday psychotherapy. During brief treatment the obsessive–compulsive and passive–dependent traits which are often particularly prominent in depressed patients are best left untouched. There simply is not enough time for efforts at character change, which is always a prolonged affair. In fact, if there is evidence that the patient's primary defenses are not functioning properly, rather than changing them one wants to bring them back to their prior best level of functioning. This is particularly true of the obsessive–compulsive defenses, which support useful strivings in the direction of autonomy, self-sufficiency, and enterprise. These defenses, rather than a liability, represent a true asset and form the principal scaffolding of the patient's personality.

During brief treatment then we mainly avoid dealing with the patient's basic personality organization and with its development over the years. Rather than at the past, our attention is directed at the patient's present and, especially, at that relationship or those relationships which currently are the source of disappointment. This area should be reviewed in great detail—the more the better—in an attempt to help the patient express the significant feelings and also reach some intellectual grasp of his difficulties. Pursuing the patient's current predicament sensitively and accurately is perhaps the essential ingredient of effective brief treatment. Unfortunately, the prescription that one should diligently attend to the present is a more difficult one to follow than is generally realized. Much loose and casual talk that we have all heard in the past few years about "working in the here and now" has made this look simpler and more obvious than it actually is. It is important to keep in mind that the past, being remote, may be less problematic than the present. Patients naturally tend to avoid what is painful and easily wander off to less conflictual, more comfortable, but also less productive topics unless they are given some steady help to stay on the track.

In certain situations, particularly when loss of self-esteem has resulted from setbacks in the patient's real life, or when one is dealing with a person in a state of borderline compensation who might not tolerate an intensive investigation of his difficulties, it may be helpful to review the patient's accomplishments with him and to emphasize what is positive, healthy, and constructive in his life rather than what is negative, shameful, and guilt-laden. A recurrent problem with depressed people is that, more than anyone else, they need to feel they conform to superior standards of goodness, but for this reason they also have enormous difficulties maintaining a comfortable estimate of their worth. Ethical demands on oneself are especially high and prominent. For example, I saw some time ago a young intern who was deeply depressed and who was considering dropping out of his internship to become a mechanic like his father. Although he had graduated first in his medical school class and had always had an outstanding scholastic record, he was haunted by the thought that he did not have enough knowledge to care for the lives of patients so that every clinical decision, large and small, became a torture for him. Until he entered treatment, the only solution to his dilemma that he was able to entertain was to leave medicine altogether. Issues of this sort, which have to do with the search for perfection and goodness, are visible in every case, even though they may not necessarily stand out as dramatically as in this instance. But it is important to be aware of the existence in depressed people of a hypertrophied and very critical conscience and, side by side, of a need to sustain an idealized view of oneself. This has to do, in other words, with the issue of narcissism. Dealing with a patient's narcissism is a complex and prolonged affair. However, a useful short-term technique for increasing the patient's sense of worth is to stimulate him to talk about the things which he does well and enjoys doing. Usually these are one and the same. As the patient speaks of his accomplishments, he gradually brings forth an image of himself as a person who is at least relatively successful, and this altered self-image, which is different from the one he originally brought into the physician's office, carries with it a new sense of hope and confidence which strengthens him as he approaches the tasks that lie ahead.

A related point, which is almost too obvious to be mentioned and yet is frequently forgotten, is that the depressed person's image of himself and his circumstances inevitably is so skewed toward the negative that often it warps the person's judgment. This is true even of patients who are not psychotic. It is also important to emphasize that, because the patient genuinely feels so bad, his view of doom and gloom is presented in an extremely convincing way. But it should be clear that this view, which is presented so sincerely and earnestly, represents the patient's subjective state and not his actual circumstances. A common problem for the inexperienced therapist is that he often takes the patient's gloomy predictions at face value and ends up agreeing with them. The result is helpless frustration and, for both patient and therapist, a sense of not knowing which way to turn. As an example of this kind of problem, let me tell you about a professional man nearing 40 who presented himself deeply depressed with the conviction that he was about to be fired from his job. He felt that this would effectively put an end to his scientific career and make him unable to support his family. He made all this appear very plausible. My task fortunately was made simpler in this case because the patient happened to bring along to his initial session a copy of his curriculum vitae. This showed at a glance that he was an unusually talented, accomplished, and productive man. I thanked him for bringing the C.V. and then said to him something to the effect that I realized that his apprehensions were very serious but also that they reflected his state of mind rather than his actual circumstances. He protested, of course, that I had not understood him and had failed to grasp the gravity of his situation. However, I reaffirmed my comment and we went on from there. It is perhaps unnecessary for me to add that he was *not* fired from his job and that his career has continued to unfold successfully.

The doctor's response to the depressed patient must take into account certain crucial features of the psychopathology of depression. These include not only the tendency to gloomy and fearful expectations but also a sense of wariness and uncertainty in his relations with people. Put more simply, the depressed patient is always a very sensitive person who is much afraid of being criticized, disapproved of, or made to feel unwanted. This means that his relationship to the doctor must be managed with special care. His feelings are easily wounded by an inadvertently sharp word or even by a faint, if unintended, tone of condemnation, and he is equally put off by aggressive warmth and too-easy familiarity as he is by apparent detachment and a formal manner. The patient wants to convince himself that the physician likes him and thinks well of him, but he is made even more guarded and suspicious by anything that approaches a stereotyped show of benevolence. When the depressed patient leaves your office after the first visit, he often looks at you in a way that says that he is not sure the treatment will work out but also that he cannot wait to come back for the next appointment. He really would like to stay longer and he wishes that the hour were not yet over. He wants more. He scans you apprehensively with his eyes as he waits to see what your last words—your verdict—will be. Do you genuinely believe you can help him and, if so, is it because you can be counted on and really understand his problem or because you have naively underestimated the extent of his difficulties? The physician, in other words, needs to be especially attuned to the multiple and constantly shifting meanings of the patient's communication, which includes not only what he says but also what he does not say, the way he looks, sits down, or takes leave of you. Treating a depressed patient is always something of an exercise in alertness and there is even less room than with other patients for momentary lapses in the therapist's attention. The depressed patient particularly requires a flexible adjustment to his mood level, warm understanding, and quiet respect, attitudes which should not be confused with overkindness or reassurance. He seeks the encouragement and support which only a verbally and emotionally responsive therapist can provide, yet simple reassurance is actually taken by the patient to mean that the doctor has little grasp of his problem. Increasing the frequency of visits is one of the practical means by which one can convey a sense of greater care, involvement, and protection when the patient is especially needy and distressed, and for some patients an invitation to call you on the phone, if they need to, can be quite helpful.

In conclusion and in summary, let me review the fundamental requirements and basic steps in the brief psychotherapeutic treatment of the depressed patient.

The first task, as with any other medical condition, is to give the patient some understanding and appreciation of what is bothering him. It is remarkable how often patients come for help for a variety of depressive complaints without realizing in the least that they are, in fact, depressed. Some improvement usually comes about when this is explained to the patient and when he is told that he can be helped to get better. The second step is to obtain a more detailed understanding of what specifically he is unhappy and distressed about. This means gathering some clues about the patient's disappointment and sense of loss and then helping him to deal with these matters in a more specific way. To identify the significant losses and disappointments one turns to the history and one looks carefully at the chronology of the symptoms. One wants to know how the trouble began, in what setting, and who are the significant persons who have disappointed or rejected the patient. Which of his expectations have not been met? When all this has been identified, it is important to keep the patient talking about these issues so as to bring about full and thorough drainage of the principal feelings, especially those of bitterness and regret. With many patients this can be effectively achieved in a limited number of sessions, and it is remarkable how successful such brief treatment can be. Even when the condition is not totally resolved within a short period, one usually notes distinct lifting of the patient's mood and some definite moves toward a more constructive approach. Before concluding, let me add a few pertinent cautions and I would ask the reader to bear with me if, for the sake of conciseness, I present these to you as simple do's and don't's.

First, address yourself to the principal reactions of disappointment and avoid tinkering with the patient's basic personality, i.e., do not involve yourself in premature and haphazard efforts at character reconstruction. Respect the patient's characteristic posture and his longstanding defenses, especially those of obsessive compulsiveness. Support these rather than try to change them.

Second, the emphasis should not be solely on the problems and the negatives. Help the patient recognize his strengths and assets since typically he is so down on himself that all he is able to see are his failures and shortcomings. Recognize what is good about him at a time when he feels so bad. Help him to achieve a more balanced and realistic view of himself.

An important third point is to talk with the patient in a spontaneous, communicative, back-and-forth style. Don't let the patient monologue and don't allow the exchange to lapse into awkward and undirected silences which leave the patient wondering where to go next. Depressed patients particularly seek "feedback" and responsiveness.

Finally, and this is especially important for the beginning therapist or the occasional psychotherapist, be careful that the patient does not discourage *you* with his gloom, his pessimism, and his hopelessness. Through your own equanimity, keep the patient aware that his problems *are* soluble and that he *can* look forward to feeling better. Should the therapist need some reassurance (and even experienced therapists occasionally do) he can find some comfort by reminding himself that depression, particularly in the milder forms, tends to be self limited. In other words, generally it improves even without treatment, but it will improve faster and more decisively if the therapist provides the patient his warm, thoughtful, and perceptive attention.

REFERENCES

1. Castelnuovo-Tedesco P: Brief psychotherapy. In: Arieti, S (ed) *The American Handbook of Psychiatry.* (2nd ed.) Vol. 5, Chap. 13, pp. 254–268. New York, Basic Books, 1975.
2. Freud S: Mourning and melancholia (1917). In: Strachey J (ed) *Standard Edition.* Vol. 14, pp. 243–258. London, Hogarth, 1957.

12

Cognitive Therapy of Depressed Suicidal Outpatients

AARON T. BECK and DAVID BURNS

We have been conducting a series of studies testing the efficacy of short-term structured psychotherapy for chronically or intermittently depressed suicidal outpatients. To date we have treated over 200 depressed patients with a new psycotherapeutic approach which we call *cognitive therapy*. This approach views depression as a disorder having emotional, motivational, behavioral, and cognitive components. We find that the cognitive component involves distorted thinking which is quite accessible to intervention with a variety of techniques which will be described below. We have found that the changes in the patient's distorted cognitions have a profound effect on the emotional and behavioral components of the syndrome, resulting in significant and rapid improvement.

Our present systematic study, which involved the treatment of 44 outpatients, was designed as a controlled comparison of cognitive psycotherapy with the giving of an antidepressant drug of proven efficacy (imipramine). The sample consisted of moderately to severely depressed outpatients with relatively long histories of intermittent or chronic depression associated with suicidal ideation. Many had been hospitalized previously and all had received previous psychiatric treatment.

Patients were randomly assigned to the drug therapy ($N = 25$) or the cognitive therapy group ($N = 19$). Patients assigned to either modality were treated for 12 weeks. The patients in the cognitive therapy group were seen initially twice a week: the frequency of visits tapered off so

AARON T. BECK and DAVID BURNS • Department of Psychiatry, University of Pennsylvania School of Medicine, Philadelphia, Pennsylvania. Dr. Burns was a Fellow of the Foundations' Fund for Research in Psychiatry when this manuscript was prepared.

that the mean was 15.2 interviews for the course of treatment. Patients in the drug group were seen weekly. Imipramine was given in increasing doses to a maximum of 250 mg/day. In addition to chemotherapy, these patients received approximately 15 minutes of supportive psychotherapy at each visit.

Cognitive therapy resulted in significantly greater improvement than did imipramine on both a self-administered measure of depression (Beck Depression Inventory) and clinical ratings (Hamilton Rating Scale for Depression and Raskin Scale). We found that 78.9% of the patients in cognitive therapy showed marked improvement or complete remission of symptoms as compared to 20.0% of the pharmacotherapy patients. In addition, both treatments resulted in a substantial decrease in anxiety ratings. The dropout rate was significantly greater with pharmacotherapy (8 *S*s) than with cognitive therapy (1 *S*). Even when these dropouts were eliminated from data analysis, the cognitive therapy patients showed a significantly greater improvement than the pharmacotherapy patients (see Table I).

The significance of the studies lies in the fact that for the first time we have been able to demonstrate, in a controlled study, that psychological techniques are effective in treating moderately to severely depressed suicidal outpatients. Four recent studies conducted by investigators elsewhere using similar techniques have shown the superiority of similar cognitive therapy techniques over other forms of psychotherapy, but they treated a less severely depressed group.[1-4]

Another significant feature is that this new approach works much faster than traditional methods of psychotherapy. Most of the patients started to improve in the first week, particularly in terms of suicidal

TABLE I. STATUS OF PATIENTS AT TERMINATION OF TREATMENT

	Cognitive therapy	Imipramine
Entered treatment	19	25
Remitted[a]	15	5
Partially remitted[b]	2	7
Unremitted[c]	1	5
Dropped-out	1	8

[a]Remitted: BDI is 9 or less.
[b]Partially remitted: BDI between 10 and 15.
[c]Unremitted: BDI is 16 or above.

ideation. If our findings are replicated, a patient who receives the newer type of psychotherapy can look forward to relatively prompt relief rather than the many weeks of suffering and flirting with suicide that we observe in patients receiving traditional therapy.

Finally, this approach provides an alternative to chemotherapy in the short-term treatment of depression. It is especially indicated for those patients who cannot or will not take antidepressant drugs, who prematurely discontinue drug treatment, or who do not respond to drug treatment.

NEW FEATURES OF COGNITIVE THERAPY*

How does this type of psychotherapy compare with more conventional forms of psychotherapy? Cognitive therapy differs both in the formal structure of the therapy sessions as well as in the kind of problems that are focused on. In comparison with the more traditional psycotherapies, such as psychoanalytic therapy or client-centered therapy, the cognitive therapist actively engages the patient in the treatment process. Since the depressed patient is generally lost and disorganized, the therapist helps him to organize his thinking and his behavior. We have found that the classical psychoanalytic techniques such as free association and the use of the couch sometimes adversely affect depressed patients because they encourage them to persevere in their negative thinking and dwell on their unpleasant feelings.

In contrast to psychoanalytic therapy, the content is focused on the here and now, and little attention is paid to childhood material. The major thrust is on clarifying the patient's thinking and feeling during the therapy session and between therapy sessions. We do not make interpretations of unconscious factors. Unlike psychoanalytic therapy, in which the therapist becomes the focus of a transference neurosis involving intense emotional experiences for the patient, the cognitive therapy is directed to training the patient in a number of exercises which must be done on a daily basis as homework between the sessions. The successful completion of these assignments is stressed as a major mechanism in the therapeutic process.

In contrast to behavior therapy, we concentrate more on the patient's inner experiences than on his overt behavior. These internal states consist of his thoughts, feelings, wishes, daydreams, and at-

*For a more complete description of cognitive therapy of depression see references 5 and 6.

titudes. Whereas the goal of behavior therapy is to modify overt behavior, the goal of cognitive therapy is to change maladaptive thinking patterns. However, certain behavioral techniques are also used, and the two approaches are not mutually exclusive.

THINKING DISORDER IN DEPRESSION

Traditionally, depression has been viewed as an affective disorder pure and simple and any thinking abnormalities have been regarded as a result of the affective disturbance. In recent years, however, we have collected a considerable amount of evidence that indicates that there is a thinking disorder in depression and that this thinking disorder may be more central than was previously believed. This hypothesis has been supported by a number of clinical and experimental studies in our own research center going back almost 20 years, as well as by investigators working elsewhere.[5] For example, recent studies of the performance of depressed patients on a proverb interpretation test indicate that such individuals have a loss of abstract thinking just as schizophrenics do, although the degree of the difficulty was not as profound in the depressed group.[7] In contrast to the highly generalized and bizarre thinking of schizophrenics, the thought disorder in depression tends to be more focalized and discrete and less bizarre.

In addition to thinking in an overly concrete manner, depressives tend to have a number of other distorted or maladaptive thinking patterns. Such individuals tend to think, for example, in an all-or-nothing manner. They see the world as either black or white (dichotomous thinking). Other thinking errors in depressives include overgeneralization and selective abstraction. For example, depressed patients typically focus on the negative in the environment and overlook or discount the positive. This distorted thinking can reach delusional proportions in individuals with a severe degree of depression.

For example, a 52-year-old president of a shirt-manufacturing firm was recently referred to our clinic with an agitated depression of acute onset. He had been unable to sleep for several days and had been pacing constantly at home. At the time of initial evaluation, he was exceptionally depressed and was so agitated he was unable to sit in the chair during the interview. When he was asked the reason for his depression, he replied:

> I am a total failure as a businessman, and my company is doomed . . . essentially, we attended the wrong trade show on the West Coast five years ago. In previous years, we had gone to another show which was scheduled in New York at the same time, but I suggested we switch and go to the West Coast show instead. . . . This was a tragic mistake, and our company is in a hopeless state . . . the employees are in rags.

However, according to his wife, his partners were convinced that going to the West Coast show was one reason for the company's booming success during the past five years. In fact, they had shown a very high profit during these years. She emphasized there were no business difficulties of a serious nature, although there had been a temporary slowdown in 1976.

Because the depressed individual has a high degree of belief in his distorted cognitions, such thinking results in disturbed feelings and maladaptive behavior, which interact in a self-perpetuating system. For example, consider the businessman's all-or-nothing statement: "I have totally ruined my business and there is *no hope.* I am a complete failure in life." Any individual who believes such thoughts will experience intense feelings of sadness and despair. These feelings are taken by the patient as evidence that his negative thoughts must be accurate. When the businessman was asked what evidence there was that he was a failure, he replied: "I *feel* like a failure, therefore, I must *be* a failure. I *feel* inadequate, therefore, I must *be* inadequate. . . ."

The sense of futility and hopelessness then leads to maladaptive behavior as the depressed individual takes action based on his distorted beliefs. For example, the businessman in question becomes socially isolated because of his thought: "What's the use? My friends and the company would be better off without me." Such social withdrawal results in a decrease in positive input from the environment, including the pleasure of social interaction from friends and associates. In addition, the businessman's failure to assume his normal leadership role at his company could eventually result in adverse consequences, such as a further business slowdown. This negative input then seems to confirm the patient's prediction that the company is doomed. He does not see that he is involved in a self-fulfilling prophecy.

Essentially, we believe that depressive illness involves a vicious cycle in which cognitive distortions, negative affective experience, and maladaptive behavior become mutually reinforcing, resulting in a self-perpetuating closed system. The underlying theme of the businessman's distorted thinking is typical of many depressives and involves a negative

view of the self and the outside world, as well as the past, present, and future. Our clinical experience indicates that, as a result of such cognitive distortions, the patient feels worse, and, when he learns to correct the errors in his thinking, he feels better.

DESCRIPTION OF COGNITIVE THERAPY

The therapy we have used is directed at the "eye of the storm"—not at the patient's inner turbulence, sadness, and agitation (although they are important) but at the way he *sees* himself and his world. In brief, we attempt to identify the negative concepts and to help the patient correct them. We encourage the patient to think more realistically and, as he sees the future more objectively and views himself and his external environment with more perspective, there is a corresponding improvement in the rest of his symptomatology. The main targets of cognitive therapy involve the conceptual and behavioral aspects of the disorder. Thus, the therapy takes two forms.

1. *Behavioral:* Change irrational ideas by changing behavior. We have found that by helping the patient to resume a more productive form of behavior, there is often a corresponding change in his attitudes about himself. As he becomes more normal, he feels more normal.

The behavioral method consists of using real-life experiences to demonstrate to the patient that his negative self-concept and negative predictions about the future are incorrect. This method may take such a homely form as assigning a specific goal, having the patient make a prediction whether he will succeed (he usually expects to fail), and then carrying out the experiment. Of course, it is essential that the experiment be designed in such a way that the experimenter will know that the patient will succeed. For instance, take a patient who spends most of his time in bed. When the therapist suggests that he attempt to walk over to the day room, the patient states, "I can't do it" or "I don't have enough energy" or "I'm too weak" or "I will feel worse if I try." The therapist can engage the patient's attention in attempting to disconfirm this notion by asking him how far he thinks he can walk. The patient might say, for instance, "Just a few feet." The therapist suggests that they experiment to see whether he can walk further than he had expected. This experiment helps to undermine his fixed belief that he is too weak or deteriorated or fatigued to engage in any physical activity. After several trials of increasing distance, the patient may be able to walk around the ward, go over to the Coke machine, and reward himself with a soda. By the next day, the patient is playing ping-pong and mingling with the other patients on the ward.

2. *Verbal:* The second class of techniques is predominantly verbal; that is, we train the patient to verbalize his cognitive distortions and to apply appropriate tests to determine whether they are valid. Once the patient is able to pinpoint his erroneous ideas, we show him how to substitute more realistic and reasonable interpretations.

This overall strategy of the behavioral/verbal approach is (a) to uncover the patient's distortions; (b) to assess the degree of the patient's belief in his distortions; (c) through specifically designed experiences or logical demonstration, to show the patient the fallacy; and (d) to substitute more correct appraisals and interpretations.

We will illustrate the application of a number of these principles by demonstrating how we approach some of the problems commonly encountered in suicidal patients, including hopelessness, a sense of failure, and intense feelings of guilt. Suicidal wishes are a very prevalent and serious problem in our depressed patients. The first case illustrates the use of an unusual method to break through in an especially difficult, refractory case.

Problem: Suicidal Impulses

Many of our research studies have shown that the most crucial psychological factor in generating suicidal wishes is the patient's *hopelessness.*[8] He sees himself as trapped in a situation in which there is no exit. Because he believes his problems are insoluble, and since he views further suffering as unbearable, he therefore thinks of suicide as the only way of escaping. In dealing with such suicidal patients, we attempt to expose the patient's hopelessness as soon as possible and then to demonstrate the degree of illogical thinking and overgeneralization that goes into the hopeless thinking.

A 25-year-old married housewife was referred to the clinic for consultation because of a 5-year history of severe intractable depression with 2 years of recurrent suicide attempts, numerous episodes of self-mutilation with razor blades requiring multiple hospitalizations, and continuous closed-ward confinement for the previous 3 months. She had not responded to several years of continuous intensive analytically oriented psychotherapy, and the recommendation of the referring psychiatrist was for indefinite long-term hospitalization. At the initial evaluation, her depression ratings on the Beck Depression Inventory (38) and the Hamilton Depression Scale (24) were in the severe range and her score on a test designed to measure the degree of hopelessness was unusually high, consistent with her profound belief that her life was not worth living, that her problems were insurmountable, and that her case was hopeless. The therapist used a modified version of role playing in which she was to imagine that two attorneys were arguing her case in court. She, as the prosecutor, would try to convince the therapist that she deserved a sentence of death. The therapist, as the defense attorney, would challenge the validity of every accusation of the prosecution.

PATIENT (AS PROSECUTOR): For this patient, suicide would be an escape from life.

THERAPIST (AS DEFENSE): That argument could apply to anyone in the world. By itself, it is not a convincing reason to die.

PATIENT: The prosecutor replies the patient's life is so miserable she cannot stand it.

THERAPIST: The patient has been able to stand it up until now and maybe she can stand it a while longer. She was not always miserable in the past, and there is not proof that she will always be miserable in the future.

PATIENT: The prosecutor points out that her life is a burden to her family.

THERAPIST: The defense emphasizes that suicide will not solve this problem, since her death by suicide may prove to be a greater burden.

PATIENT: But she is self-centered and lazy.

THERAPIST: What percent of the population is lazy?

PATIENT: Probably 20%. . . . No, I'd say only 10%.

THERAPIST: That means 20 million Americans are lazy. The defense points out that they don't have to die for this, so there is no reason the patient should be singled out for death. Do you think laziness and apathy are symptoms of depression?

PATIENT: Probably.

THERAPIST: The defense points out that individuals in our culture are not sentenced to death for symptoms of an illness. Furthermore, the laziness may disappear when depression goes away.

The patient appeared involved in and amused by this repartée. After a series of such "accusations" and "defenses," she concluded that there was no convincing reason that she should have to die and that any reasonable jury would rule in favor of the defense. What was more important was that she then began to challenge and answer the negative thoughts herself, and this brought immediate emotional relief, the first she had experienced in many months. At the end of the therapy session, she said, "I have the thought: 'This new therapy may not prove to be as good as it seems'—and the answer to that is—if it isn't, I'll find out in a few weeks, and I'll still have the alternative of long-term hospitalization so I have lost nothing. Furthermore, it may be partially as good as it seems, or conceivably even better."

Although such a technique may not be curative in itself, it can provide symptomatic relief in the early phases of the treatment of the depression when suicidal impulses are particularly threatening, thus laying the groundwork for more fundamental changes in later sessions.

Problem: Sense of Failure

The second case, like the first, illustrates an unusual, somewhat dramatic technique which we sometimes use when traditional supportive methods have failed. Many patients complain of a sense of inadequacy and failure and have the conviction that they have failed as human beings. Such feelings are particularly common to suicidal patients.

A middle-aged married immigrant was brought to our clinic by her family one day after her discharge from an intensive-care unit where she had been treated for an unexpected suicide attempt. Her cognitions were focused on the idea that her life had not reached the degree of fulfillment she had dreamed of as a girl. In particular, she believed she had accomplished nothing in her life and had concluded that her life was not worth living. The therapist asked her to make a list of things she had accomplished, as a way of testing this hypothesis.

Patient: I learned to speak five languages fluently, I helped my family survive Nazi terrorism and relocate in a new country, I worked 25 years at a dreary job so more money would be available for my family, I raised a lovely son who went to college and is a success, I cook well, and my grandchildren seem to think I'm a good grandmother.

Therapist: So how can you say you have accomplished nothing?

Patient: You see, *everyone* in my family spoke five languages, getting out of Europe was *just a matter of survival,* my job required *no talent,* it is the *duty* of a mother to raise her family, and a housewife *should* learn to cook, so these are *not real accomplishments.* All this just proves that life is not worthwhile.

It seemed to the therapist that the patient was arbitrarily saying, "It doesn't count," with regard to anything good about herself. In order to demonstrate this to her, the therapist proposed they switch doctor–patient roles, in which the therapist would assume the role of himself as a patient and she would cast herself in the role of therapist.

PATIENT (IN ROLE OF THERAPIST): I understand you feel you have accomplished nothing. But you must have accomplished something.

THERAPIST (IN ROLE OF DEPRESSED PSYCHIATRIST): I care for many sick patients and I publish the results of my research.

PATIENT (IN ROLE OF THERAPIST): It sounds like you have accomplished a great deal at such a young age.

THERAPIST (IN ROLE OF DEPRESSED PSYCHIATRIST): No, it is the *obligation* of every doctor to care for his patients, and it is my *duty* in the university to do research. So these are not real accomplishments. My life is basically a failure.

PATIENT (AS HERSELF, LAUGHING): I see that I've been criticizing myself like that for the past ten years.

THERAPIST: Now, how does it feel when you say those negative things to yourself?

PATIENT: I feel depressed when I say these things.

At this point, she was able to see that she had been needlessly upsetting herself by her self-statements. When she recognized the arbitrary nature of her self-punitive statements, she experienced immediate relief of her depression as well as of the urge to commit suicide. She realized that there was no convincing evidence to support her belief that she had accomplished nothing in life. It is notable that in this case the evocation of amusement also appeared to provide greater objectivity.

PROBLEM: GUILT

A third problem often encountered in depressed suicidal patients is an intense feeling of guilt for some real or imagined wrongdoing. Such feelings are frequently based on misconceptions. The following case is of particular interest, because it deals with the problem of guilt often faced by psychiatrists when their patient commits suicide.

A 40-year-old pediatrician was referred for a severe depression of six weeks' duration following the successful suicide of her younger brother. He had been under psychiatric care for several years because of several previous nearly successful suicide attempts and she had provided him with substantial ongoing emotional and financial support. He was a physiology student and had requested information from her on the day of his death concerning the effects of carbon monoxide in the blood. He stated he needed this information for a "talk" he was to give in school, and then he used the information in his suicide, which he committed outside her apartment. She held herself responsible for his death and was seriously considering suicide.

Her depression, as measured by the Beck Depression Inventory, remained in the very severe range (32–35) until the fifth therapy session. On this day, she outlined the reasons why she felt she'd be better off dead: "I had assumed responsibility for my brother, and thus I must have failed to provide adequate support. . . . I failed to intervene when I should have known it was an acute situation. I was angry with him on the day he died and on several occasions during the previous month. At times I might even have thought he'd be better off dead. I failed, and I, too, deserve to die."

The therapist discussed the possible misconceptions in her point of view. First, he pointed out that scientists do not know for certain why people commit suicide. Since we do not know the cause of suicide, it is arbitrary to assume that *she* was the cause of his suicide. If we had to guess at the immediate cause, it would be his own convictions that he was no good and that his life was not worth living. But since she did not control his thoughts, she could not have been responsible for his mental error. This was his error and not hers. Finally, she did not have the knowledge necessary to prevent his death, just as she did not always have the proper knowledge to save the life of every cancer patient she treated. But if she did have such knowledge to help her brother, she certainly would have used it. Her error consisted in holding herself responsible for his behavior. She could try to help him but she could not expect herself to control his behavior.

She expressed the idea at this point that she was *not* responsible for his suicide, but rather he had been. She, in fact, was responsible for her own life and well-being. She also mused that she was acting irresponsibly with regard to her own life by considering ways of killing herself.

This discussion was followed by a rapid remission of the depression over the next three sessions, which the patient attributed to a "cognitive switch" which resulted from exposing her misconceptions that she had been the cause of her brother's suicide and was responsible for his death. She then elected to remain in therapy to work on the problem of chronic depression which she had experienced for many years.

The rationale of these particular therapeutic interventions is based on the concept that the depressed patient has arrived at an erroneous belief about himself and his future. He does not even think to question the belief. Even when contradicting data are presented, he may hold on to it. However, by introducing "cognitive dissonance," i.e., by inducing the patient to look at the inner contradiction in his belief, we open up this closed system to corrective information. In essence, the thrust of the therapy is to improve the patient's reality testing.

In summary, our cognitive techniques consist of (1) helping the patient to identify his negative thinking, (2) getting him to examine his cognitions and determine the overgeneralizations, selective abstractions, and exaggerations, (3) bringing the weight of evidence into play, and (4) helping him to reinterpret his experiences in a more realistic way.

We have found that, once the patient starts to interpret life situations more accurately, there tends to be a change in the cycle of depression: Realistic cognitions, increased hope and self-esteem, and more appropriate behavior begin to interact in a positively reinforcing system.

New Directions for Research

Our research indicates that cognitive therapy can be effective in the treatment of depressed outpatients. We would like to emphasize that this was a preliminary study and that further studies will be required to confirm these findings with a larger patient sample and to determine the general applicability of our findings. If further studies are consistent with the initial findings, we will be interested in exploring the question: What makes this therapy effective? To what extent are the specific techniques, as opposed to the therapists' enthusiasm, confidence, and emphasis on hope, important factors which result in change?

A second area of interest involves the rapid switch process out of depression which sometimes occurs in the course of a therapy session. We have observed this change in a significant number of patients, such as the pediatrician described earlier. What cognitive changes are occurring during these therapy sessions, and what therapeutic interventions facilitate those rapid reversals in mood?

A third question concerns the interaction between psychopharmacology and cognitive therapy. We are currently evaluating the hypothesis that these two approaches will be additive and that the combination of drug therapy and cognitive therapy may provide more rapid relief than either approach alone.

Our long-range plan is to determine what forms of treatment are most effective for specific subgroups of depression. In this way we will be able to fit the treatment to the patient and provide a more rational basis for prescriptive therapy.

REFERENCES

1. Taylor FG, Marshall WL: Experimental analysis of a cognitive-behavioral therapy for depression. *Cognitive Therapy and Research 1:*59–72, 1977.
2. Shaw BF: Comparison of cognitive therapy and behavior therapy in the treatment of depression. *J. Consult. Clin. Psychol. 45:*543–551, 1977.
3. Morris NE: A group self-instruction method for the treatment of depressed outpatients. Unpublished doctoral dissertation, University of Toronto, 1975.
4. Schmickley VG: The effects of cognitive-behavior modification upon depressed outpatients. Unpublished doctoral dissertation, Michigan State University, 1976.
5. Beck AT: *Depression: Causes and Treatment.* Philadelphia, University of Pennsylvania Press, 1972.
6. Beck AT: *Cognitive Therapy and the Emotional Disorders.* New York, International Universities Press, 1976.
7. Braff DL, Beck AT: Thinking disorder in depression. *Arch. Gen. Psychiatry 31:*456–459, 1974.
8. Beck AT, Kovacs M, Weissman A: Hopelessness and suicidal behavior: An overview. *JAMA 234:*1146–1149, 1975.
9. Rush AJ, Beck AT, Kovacs M, Hollon S: Comparative efficacy of cognitive therapy and pharmacotherapy in the treatment of depressed outpatients. *Cognitive Therapy and Research 1:*17–37, 1977.

13

Combining Drugs and Psychotherapy in the Treatment of Depression

GERALD L. KLERMAN

The chapters in this volume are typical of the current therapeutic approach in American psychiatry. Treatment is pluralistic, and the theoretical approach eclectic. Practitioners mix drug treatment with various kinds of psychotherapy—cognitive, psychoanalytic, or behavioral; group or family. Occasionally electroconvulsive therapy (ECT) is prescribed.

Although the therapeutic approach is practical, the theoretical rationale for these practices is seldom articulated. American psychiatry continues to be involved in theoretical discussions based on the mind–body dualism. The question arises whether there is any way to relate these various treatments to a body of scientific theory. American psychiatry will continue to be a "split-brain preparation": one half exploring the psyche with the other half exploring the soma.

In this paper I will analyze the basis for combining drugs and psychotherapy in depression. In practice, most depressed patients are treated with some combination of drugs and individual psychotherapy. There are, however, important exceptions where drugs or psychotherapy are used alone. In this chapter, I will attempt to develop a comprehensive understanding of these three alternatives.

In combining treatments the problem facing the psychiatrist is similar to that of the bartender. In practice, psychiatrists are mixing various therapeutic "cocktails." Family therapy is mixed with Elavil or group therapy combined with Thorazine. Like the martini, where gin and ver-

GERALD L. KLERMAN • Stanley Cobb Psychiatric Research Laboratories, Psychiatry Service, Massachusetts General Hospital, and Department of Psychiatry, Harvard Medical School, Boston, Massachusetts.

mouth have been found to potentiate one another, the assumption in psychiatric treatment "cocktails" is that the ingredients will "go well together"—that is, that they will have additive or even synergistic effects. Thus the goal and method of combined treatment is essentially the same as that which the bartender pursues, attempting to generate "cocktails." A bartender works by trial and error, as has also psychiatric therapeutic practice, it appears. Lately, however, there has been a growing body of research on evaluation of treatments: drug treatment has been widely researched; the quantity and quality of psychotherapeutic research has improved; and there is a small but growing body of research on combined treatments.

Reviewing the situation, I have divided the proponents of the alternative approaches into three groups: (1) the proponents of drug treatment, i.e., those who "like their drinks straight"; (2) the proponents of psychotherapy, i.e., those who are "prohibitionists"; (3) the proponents of combined therapy, i.e., those who are seeking psychiatric–therapeutic "cocktails." In this discussion, I will examine each of these three alternative approaches in some detail.

THE PROPONENTS OF DRUG THERAPY—OR THOSE WHO LIKE THEIR DRINKS STRAIGHT

While at first glance combined treatment, or cocktails, would seem self-evidently reasonable, there is an important group of psychiatrists who do not accept combined treatment but who emphasize the importance of drug treatment. They "like their drinks straight." Their view is that drugs are the necessary and perhaps even sufficient ingredient in treatment—all that the patient needs. Some propose that other forms of treatment are at times unnecessary, expensive, and disruptive.

While the assumption with most cocktails is that the combination is positively additive, some members of this group of psychiatrists argue that combining psychotherapy and drugs produces a negative effect. Psychotherapy may "stir the patient up" by discussing childhood memories or current conflicts and thus may increase the state of psychophysiological arousal—for example, by stimulating adrenocortical or sympathetic activity. Their contention is that this increased physiological arousal goes against the pharmacological effects of the drugs.

This group of psychiatrists argues that there is a direct relationship between the introduction of modern drug therapy and the improvements in the treatment of the mentally ill and, among depressives, in particular in the treatment of those hospitalized with psychotic depressions yet also of the ambulatory or psychoneurotic depressives. This view has been most widely held by mental health professionals working in public mental health institutions with severely ill patients and is also held by a large number of practitioners in private practice and outpatient clinics. They belong to what Hollingshead and Redlich identified as the Directive and Organic (D & O) group of practitioners.[1] However, they most often call themselves *biological psychiatrists*. These psychiatrists, along with many journalists and public officials, have concluded that these new drugs not only improved patient treatment but brought about a revolution in psychiatry, returning psychiatry to the "mainstream" of modern medicine. Many supporters of drug therapy have an implicit, and at times explicit, antipsychotherapeutic bias and regard the success of drug therapy as support for their long-held criticism of Freudianism and related psychotherapeutic theories.

Among those involved in the treatment of depressions, proponents of this point of view included many previous advocates of ECT and the strong enthusiasts for lithium, who often combined their support of ECT and drug therapies with criticism of psychotherapy as valueless, unproven as to efficacy, or harmful.

During discussions in the 1940s and 1950s, the psychotherapists were the aggressive parties to the dialogue and the biological therapists were on the defensive; since the 1960s there has been a significant shift in favor of biological psychiatry. Considering the demonstrated efficacy of drugs for the treatment of depression and the relatively smaller body of evidence for the efficacy of psychotherapy, the question has been stated: What benefit accrues to the depressed patient through psychotherapy added upon drug therapy?

At least three component views can be identified among the biological psychiatrists.

Psychotherapy May Be Symptomatically Disruptive

Some psychiatrists state that psychotherapy is deleterious to drug treatment since symptoms may be aggravated. These psychiatrists who have worked with drug treatment for depressives and schizophrenics feel that harm may be done to the patient by psychotherapeutic intervention, particularly during the acute illness, and that the patient is best left alone to "heal over" and to reconstitute. There is a conflict between those psychiatrists who advocate working through underlying conflicts in depression and others who support healing or sealing over by promoting denial, repression, and other defenses. The situation hypothesized by many pharmacotherapists is that psychotherapy, by uncovering areas of conflict, will increase the levels of tension or arousal.

Drugs as Biochemical Replacement

Most biological psychiatrists compare psychiatric drug treatment to use of drugs used in general medicine, especially to agents like insulin for diabetes. This view argues that drug treatment alone is necessary and sufficient. For those who hold this view, the rectification by drugs of the presumed neurophysiological dysfunction or biochemical deficiency is the critical therapeutic factor, and psychotherapy is considered unnecessary and irrelevant or, at best, neutral. A variation of this is expressed by some proponents of lithium treatment for recurrent depression.

Psychotherapy as Rehabilitation

In practice, however, most drug therapists accept some form of psychotherapy, but as secondary and ameliorative therapy. They believe psychotherapy operates not upon etiological mechanisms at the core of the depressive illness process but only to correct secondary difficulties in interpersonal relations, self-esteem, and psychologic functions that follow upon the impact of depressive symptoms. In this view psychotherapy is rehabilitative rather than therapeutic in the classical medical model. As such, it would be an elective rather than a necessary component of the treatment program.

Having identified these three variants of the views of proponents of drug therapy, I would like to comment on some sources of the controversy.

Part of the disagreement may be due to the types of patients the different classes of therapists see. The biological psychiatrist focuses attention on the bipolar and recurrent unipolar types of affective disorder. However, it is important to realize that, while these types may respond significantly to medication, they afflict a minority of depressed patients, at most 20% to 30%. The vast majority of depressions are not bipolar and are variously called *neurotic, secondary, reactive,* or other vague diagnostic terms. It may well be that for these classes of patients the drugs we use have a relatively nonspecific effect compared to the effects of lithium on bipolar patients. It may be also that for such patients an environmental or social stress has played an important role in the precipitation of reactive or neurotic depressions. This provides more of a rationale for the psychotherapeutic approach, whether used alone or in combination with drugs.

There is limited evidence for the disruptive effect of psychotherapy on drug therapy in depression. It may well be that, in some forms of endogenous depression and in bipolar types of manic-depression, treatment with lithium or tricyclics is the major ingredient and that the psychotherapy has only limited added benefit. As such, it would be as a form of rehabilitation, to assist recovery promoted by the drug, rather than as something specific or necessary.

The bipolar type of manic-depressive illness has been the focus of considerable attention, particularly in biological research. Yet it constitutes only about 10% of all depressed patients. The bread and butter of clinical psychiatry is the so-called *neurotic* or *reactive* depressive, who is neither unipolar nor bipolar. This patient usually has associated personality and character problems and difficult life circumstances, and his/her family conflicts and maladaptive life style often go back to childhood. The existence of this large group has sustained attention to the importance of psychotherapy and supported the proponents of psychotherapy.

THE PROPONENTS OF PSYCHOTHERAPY— "THE PROHIBITIONISTS"

At the opposite end of the theoretical and therapeutic spectrum from the biological psychiatrists are the proponents of psychotherapy. I call them "prohibitionists" because they do not want to use any medicinal agents.

The prohibitionists are less influential than they were ten years ago, but they are nevertheless an important part of psychiatric practice and even more in psychotherapeutic practice conducted by nonphysicians. Some argue that psychotherapy is all that is necessary. Others argue that drug therapy will undermine the transference and countertransference reactions and promote the patients' dependency needs. They believe these effects to be due to the prescription of the drug *per se,* even if it is a placebo, let alone an active drug. An important component of their argument implies a variant of the negative placebo effect, as will be discussed—namely, that the writing of the prescription and the ingestion of the pill has the effect of undermining the doctor–patient relationship and is deleterious for the outcome of psychotherapy.

Some psychotherapists are skeptical of the evidence for the value of drugs in depression. These skeptics are comprised mainly of private practitioners skilled in psychotherapy, many clinical psychologists, and a large group of social psychologists and researchers who question whether the antidepressant drugs have a "real" effect at all. The skeptics point to the newfound enthusiasm and therapeutic zeal enunciated by the pharmacologic prescribers and wonder whether a placebo effect and the Hawthorne effect are perhaps the significant source of the claimed efficacy of drugs. Psychiatry, it is noted, has witnessed previous periods of enthusiasm and optimism for new treatments back through mesmerism in the eighteenth century and numerous other fads for both psychic and somatic treatments. The skeptics point to the extensive research in industrial settings on the Hawthorne effect, whereby any increase in attention and attitudinal enthusiasm had a positive effect on a group situation, ameliorating conflict and increasing the productivity of workers. They propose that similar enthusiasm and attention on the part of psychiatrists who were previously pessimistic and nihilistic are being communicated to patients and their families. This Hawthorne effect would interact with the placebo effect to enhance the patient's participation, interacting still further with the zeal and enthusiasm of the physician. This would bring into question whether or not the therapeutic benefits attributed to antidepressant drugs are in fact due to these social–psychological forces rather than the pharmacologic actions of the drugs upon the central nervous system.

While the skeptics have raised questions as to the efficacy of drugs, other more radical critics have been openly derogatory of them. They suggest that not only are the drugs little more than placebos but more importantly that they are actually detrimental to the patient's welfare and have adverse effects not only upon the patient but upon the psychiatrist and the family. Drug therapy impairs the patient's progress in psychotherapy, increasing his/her magical reliance upon biological treatment, fostering dependency upon the physician, and blunting capacity for insight. In addition to these deleterious effects upon patients, opponents regard the new tranquilizing and antidepressant drugs as having harmful effects on psychotherapists, limiting their skills by encouraging tendencies to seek quick, ready solutions to complex problems. Similar concerns are expressed about the effect upon the family, tempting them to look to drug treatment as support for explaining the patient's illness in terms of "nerves" and "real" illness rather than having to look to conflict, guilt, and other psychological issues which may involve personal responsibility and the need for change in lifestyle or family practices. The radical critics have challenged the medical model for its being authoritarian and biological and assert that in prescribing drugs physicians are using chemical straightjackets or participating in the maintenance of conformity in a repressive society.[2,3]

In regard to drug treatment of depression, the radical feminist movement most strongly expresses this prohibitionist view. Pharmacotherapy hinders "feminist" liberation, it is argued, because it regards the depressed woman's problems as biomedical and deflects the depressed woman's attention from consciousness-raising efforts and, ultimately,from social change to end sexism and promote equality.

Among the large group of prohibitionists it is possible to discern a number of component views.

The Negative Placebo Effect

Much of the criticism of drug therapy enunciated by psychotherapists implies negative placebo effect, that medication has harmful effects on psychotherapy. It is claimed that the prescription of any drug has active or inactive deleterious effects upon the psychotherapeutic relationship and upon the attitudes and behavior of both patient and therapist—effects independent of the specific pharmacologic actions of the drug. In addition, critics feel the prescription of medications promotes an authoritarian attitude on the part of the psychiatrist, enhancing belief in his/her biological–medical heritage. At the same time, the patient becomes more dependent, places greater reliance on magical thinking, and assumes a more passive, compliant role in fields of medicine other than psychiatry. Drug treatment is feared to be initiating and/or augmenting of countertransference and transference processes which run counter to the development of insight and the uncovering of defenses.

Drug Induced Reduction of Anxiety and Symptoms as a Motive for Discontinuing or Avoiding Psychotherapy

In contrast to the negative placebo effect noted above, which deals with only the symbolic and psychological meaning of drug administration, another critical view acknowledges the pharmacologic and therapeutic actions of drugs but expresses concern that the resultant drug-induced decrease of a patient's anxiety and tension will reduce motivation for psychotherapeutic participation. This hypothesis predicts that too-effective drug action initiates forces operating counter to the patient's progress in psychotherapy. Thus, if a psychoactive drug, such as a tricyclic or a diazepoxide derivative, is highly effective in reducing depression, the patient's motivation for reflection, insight, and psychotherapeutic work will be lessened.[2,3] In this view it is predicted that, if drug therapy is too effective, patients will no longer seek psychotherapy because they will be satisfied with symptom reduction and, therefore, cease working towards deeper personality, characterologic, or social change. The radical feminist critique embodies this point of view.

Possible Deleterious Effects of Pharmacotherapy upon Psychotherapy Expectations

There may be a negative reaction among some patients for whom drug therapy is prescribed instead of psychotherapy. Such patients may feel that the prescription of a drug defines them as "less interesting" and as unsuitable candidates for insight. Thus, the psychiatrist's prescription of drugs may be interpreted by the patient as loss of status, especially if he/she belongs to a subculture whose values emphasize insight, psychotherapeutic understanding, and self-actualization. This expectation varies with the social class and subculture in which the patient participates. Within groups that value psychotherapy, the use of drugs is often regarded as a "failure" or "crutch."

Over the past decade, many of the fears expressed by the prohibitionists concerning drug therapy have not materialized. There is little evidence for negative placebo effect. There has been no marked reduction in the public's overall utilization of psychotherapy; in fact, the public's confidence in psychiatry and mental health services continues to grow.

The primacy of psychotherapy in specific clinical situations has diminished, especially in schizophrenia, other major psychoses, mania, and severe depressions. In psychiatric practice, a major rapprochement appears to have occurred. The majority of medically trained psychotherapists are increasingly comfortable about use of drugs. Only a small minority remains prohibitionist. However, among the growing numbers of nonmedical psychotherapists, social workers, and others hesitant, ambivalent, or negative attitudes toward drug therapy seem to exist.

THE PRAGMATIC COMBINERS OF DRUGS AND PSYCHOTHERAPY—"THE COCKTAIL MIXERS"

In practice, most psychiatrists and even many nonmedical psychotherapists are active bartenders, mixing various "cocktails" of drugs and psychotherapy. The largest group of practitioners are eclectic and pragmatic. Whatever may have been their theoretical orientation, in practice they prescribe drugs with increasing frequency. They often combine drugs with psychotherapy on a trial-and-error basis. However, the theoretical justifications for this practice remain vague and weak.

When we ask psychiatrists to explain their rationales for prescribing various therapies for depression, we can identify inconsistent responses. If we ask a psychotherapeutically oriented psychiatrist why he/she uses a particular psychotherapeutic technique, he/she will almost always answer in concepts and terms derived from psychodynamic theory, e.g., resolution of conflict, etc.

In prescribing drugs in combination with psychotherapy for depression, psychiatrists expect that the drugs will reduce manifest symptoms and lower the subjective distress of the patients. Prominent symptoms, such as anxiety, insomnia, tension, and autonomic manifestations, become the target symptoms for drug prescription. The psychiatrist expects the drugs to reduce the patient's subjective distress and hopes thereby to facilitate communication, to reduce resistance to therapeutic insight, and to accelerate psychotherapeutic progress. This pragmatic view assumes that both treatments are effective and, furthermore, that the combination will have a positive interaction—additive, and even hopefully synergistic. The rationales for mixing this cocktail can be analyzed into two basic forms: (1) the two-stage treatment strategy and (2) the facilitation of psychotherapeutic accessibility.

The Two-Stage Treatment Strategy

A very common rationale for the use of drugs and psychotherapy in combination involves a two-stage treatment strategy in which a drug or ECT is used to reduce disturbance or excitation in the initial phase; following this, in the second stage, psychotherapy is relied upon most. This strategy most often is applied for very disturbed patients, severe endogenous depressions, psychotic depressions, or manic-depressive types of affective disorders in the acute manic or depressive phase. Drug treatment or ECT is prescribed to assist the patient over the acute stage, when symptoms may be distressing or disturbing. Psychotherapy during this stage is used mainly for supportive purposes and for establishing a relationship for future long-term goals. During this first stage there is exploration of topics, to develop the "agenda," so-to-speak, for the psychotherapeutic work. In part, this strategy depends on differences in the kinetics of the two treatments. Drug treatment tends to work quickly and to be effective primarily against symptom formation. Psychotherapy, however, may have a slower onset and a longer latency; the targets for its efficacy are primarily interpersonal relations, social adjustment, and personal competence of the patient and less often symptom reduction. Thus, the combination of drugs and psychotherapy is useful in two ways; drugs and psychotherapy operate at two different stages in the treatment process and upon two different targets.

In this respect, the "cocktail" is like a two-stage rocket. The first stage of the rocket, i.e., drugs, gets the patient "out of the symptomatic orbit" or "out of the gravity field" of symptomatology; and then in the second stage the psychotherapy puts him/her into the realm of social adjustment, personal competence, and perhaps even insight.

Facilitation of Psychotherapeutic Accessibility

Advertisements and other promotional materials of many pharmaceutical firms propose that the introduction of their drug facilitates psychotherapy by making the patient "more accessible." The proposed mechanism for this facilitating effect is readily specified—the pharmacologic action of the drug ameliorates the presumed CNS dysfunction underlying symptom formation, resulting in reduction of the patient's symptoms and/or affective discomfort. Drug-induced reduction in discomfort renders the patient better able to communicate in and benefit from psychotherapy. While some level of anxiety, dysphoria, or symptomatology is believed necessary to provide the "drive" or motivation for participation in psychotherapy, this hypothesis, on the other hand, presumes that excessive levels of tension, anxiety, or symptom intensity result in a decrease in the patient's capacity to participate effectively in psychotherapy.

Implicit in this rationale is a model of an inverted-U-shaped curve of the relationship between accessibility and level of symptomatic distress (Figure 1). When distress is too low, there is not enough anxiety or tension to "drive the system" and the patient is too little motivated to seek psychotherapy. However, at the right-handed end of the curve when distress is too high the patient is inaccessible to psychological influence. Most psychotic patients fall into the high end of the curve. Normal persons fall into the low end of the distress range. The ideal psychotherapeutic patient is considered to be one who lies at the midpoint—that is, has sufficient symptomatic distress to be motivated to seek psychotherapeutic assistance but is not so overwhelmed by suicidal

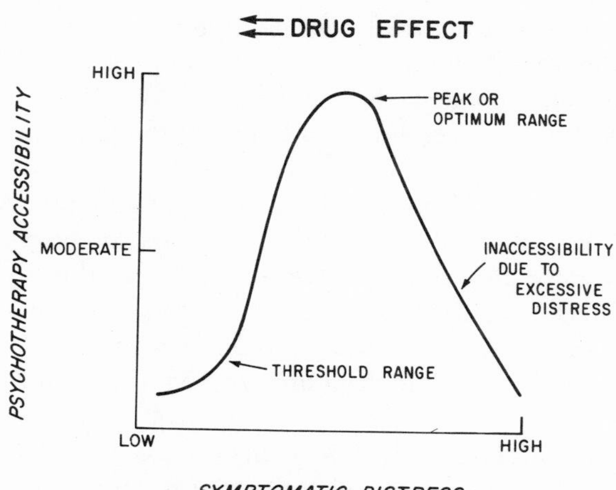

Figure 1. The action of drugs to facilitate psychotherapeutic accessibility.

drives, anxiety, guilt, or other symptoms that he/she cannot attend to the psychotherapy.

The function of drug therapy, according to this model, is to move the patient into levels of lower distress and, therefore, more accessibility. This is best exemplified by use of the phenothiazines in schizophrenia, but also by the use of tricyclics in depression. Patients who are otherwise too anxious, too guilt-ridden, too sleep-deprived or otherwise distressed to engage in psychotherapy have their symptoms sufficiently reduced. This curve is also related to the effects of anxiety upon other forms of performance such as athletic endeavor or scholastic achievement. Those psychotherapists concerned with the "flight into health" that may be prompted by drug therapy are fearful that drug therapy will move the patient too far to the left—that is, will make the patient so asymptomatic and so free of distress that he/she will feel no motivation to continue working on underlying problems or to seek psychotherapeutic help. Some variant of this inverted-U-shaped model is, in my opinion, the dominant rationale for the use of combined treatment.

The combination of drugs and psychotherapy in psychiatric treatment is widely used but inadequately understood. Ultimately, data from controlled trials will be necessary to support this therapeutic practice. These issues are currently evident in the treatment of depression where drugs and psychotherapy, the most frequently prescribed therapeutic modalities, can be related to relatively well-specified, although only partially validated, theoretical models—the neurochemical models which explain and justify drug treatment and the psychodynamic models which underlie psychotherapeutic methods. Depression, therefore, presents one area of psychiatry which is theoretically active and therapeutically successful and where linkages between theory, experiment, and practice are emerging.

The data available from the small but growing number of controlled studies demonstrate no negative interactions between drugs and psychotherapy for depression. On the contrary, there are probably synergistic effects due to the different processes that influence the two treatments. Psychotherapy seems to influence interpersonal relations and social performance while drug therapy reduces symptom formation and affective distress. There are, moreover, sequential interactions such that sustained symptom reduction seems a necessary condition for the efficacy of psychotherapy. Of all the various rationales, the one that postulates that drugs render the patient more accessible to psychotherapy is best supported by the available data.

CONCLUSIONS

Ideally, in prescribing combined treatment, the psychiatrist's decision should be based on four types of available evidence:

1. Evidence for the efficacy of each treatment alone.
2. Understanding of their respective mechanisms of action.
3. Knowledge of the efficacy of the combination.
4. Verified theory which provides a reasonable and understandable basis for the combination.

It should be acknowledged that in the use of combined drugs and psychotherapy for depression we are far from having these four types of evidence. We have many controlled studies as to the efficacy of the drugs and partially verified hypotheses as to their mode of action. There are a few controlled studies supporting the efficacy of psychotherapy in depression although there is a highly elaborated theory of the psychodynamics of depression. Concepts bridging the distance between pharmacology and psychodynamics are relatively few, and empirical studies as to the value and limitation of combined therapy are emerging but are still limited.

As stated, the ideal situation in assessing the theoretical and therapeutic aspects of combined psychotherapy and drug therapy would be to possess empirical evidence about the efficacy and safety of each of these therapies. With respect to the efficacy and safety of antidepressant drug therapy, the quantity and quality of the evidence is very favorable. Since the mid-1950s there have been a large number of controlled clinical trials which have demonstrated the efficacy of the tricyclic antidepressants, the MAO inhibitors, phenothiazines, and lithium compared with placebo or other control factors. For symptom relief and resolution of the acute depressive episode, drug therapy has demonstrated efficacy. In addition, there is now substantial evidence for the value of two classes of drugs for maintenance therapy to prevent relapse and recurrence: lithium for both bipolar and unipolar depressions and the tricyclics for unipolar recurrent depressions and various forms of neurotic depressions characterized by relapse and fluctuation.[4]

When, however, we review the psychotherapy of depression, the evidence for its efficacy is more limited but improving rapidly. The efficacy of psychotherapy is a subject of continual controversy[5]; however, there are now almost a dozen controlled studies showing the efficacy of psychotherapy for depression. Studies have been reported on individual psychotherapy done by social workers,[6] group therapy,[7] and family therapy.[8] These three studies report on therapies attempting to modify the patient's interpersonal patterns. Some newer psychotherapies are based on behaviorism, derived particularly from the research of Lewinsohn.[9] One of Lewinsohn's students, Peter McLean, has recently reported on results of a controlled trial showing the efficacy of behavioral therapy.[10] A. J. Rush and A. T. Beck have reported a pilot study on the efficacy of cognitive behavioral therapy, showing it to be equivalent to tricyclic antidepressant treatment.[11] Brian Shaw reported results of various forms of group treatment based on both cognitive and behavioral theories of depression.[12]

Evidence in support of combined treatment has only recently emerged and at a very slow pace. Luborsky et al. in a comprehensive review of controlled studies of the efficacy of psychotherapy, identified nine published studies on the combination of drugs and psychotherapy.[5] Eight of the nine studies showed efficacy of the combination over and above the individual constituents alone.

Drugs and psychotherapy derive from different theoretical realms and *a priori* should be neutral to one another, but ideologically they are in conflict. Although considerable psychophysiological research has been undertaken in animals and man to document the possible mechanisms by which conflict and stress influence brain function (particularly via pituitary, hypothalmic, and subcortical mechanisms), endocrine activity, and amine metabolism, experimentally based formulations for the use of psychotherapy combined with drug therapy are rare. Recent psychobiological studies in psychophysiology, biofeedback, and neurochemistry provide more sophisticated insights into biobehavioral interaction. It is hoped that these insights will break the theoretical mind–body dualism so tenaciously held by adherents of exclusively biological or psychotherapeutic approaches within psychology and psychiatry.

Unfortunately, in the development of scientific psychiatry, clinical practices are still ahead of systematic investigations. In most therapeutic decisions, pragmatic experience more often guides the psychiatrist than does evidence culled from systematic clinical trials, experimental studies on animals, or basic laboratory research.

The treatment of depression thus serves as only one example of the compartmentalized and fragmented state of contemporary theory and practice. In building a scientific psychiatry, the issues raised by the treatment of depression with combined drugs and psychotherapy apply equally to treatment of other clinical psychiatric states, and most of the problems described in this chapter are only specific illustrations of general problems in the theory and practice of psychiatric therapeutics.

ACKNOWLEDGMENTS

Appreciation is expressed to Alberto DiMascio, Ph.D.; Brigette Prusoff, M.P.H.; and Myrna M. Weissman, Ph.D.; my associates in the Boston–New Haven Collaborative Depression Project, for many of the ideas included in this chapter.

REFERENCES

1. Hollingshead A, Redlich F: *Social Class and Mental Illness.* New York, Wiley and Sons, 1958.
2. Szasz T: Some observations on the use of tranquilizing drugs. *Arch. Neurol. Psychiatry 77:*86, 1957.
3. Meerloo J: Medication into submission: The danger of therapeutic coercion. *J. Nerv. Ment. Dis. 122:*353, 1955.
4. Klerman G, DiMascio A, Weissman M et al.: Treatment of depression by drugs and psychotherapy. *Am. J. Psychiatry 131:*186–191, 1974.
5. Luborsky L, Singer B, Luborsky L: Comparative studies of psychotherapies. *Arch. Gen. Psychiatry 32:*995–1008, 1975.
6. Weissman M, Klerman G, Paykel E et al.: Treatment effects on the social adjustment of depressed patients. *Arch. Gen. Psychiatry 30:*771–778, 1975.
7. Covi L, Lipman R, Derogatis L et al.: Drugs and group psychotherapy in neurotic depression. *Am. J. Psychiatry 131:*191–198, 1974.
8. Friedman A et al.: Drugs and family therapy in the treatment of depression. *Arch. Gen. Psychiatry 32:*619–637, 1975.
9. Lewinsohn P: A behavioral approach to depression. In: Friedman R, Katz M (eds) *The Psychology of Depression: Contemporary Theory and Research.* Washington, D.C., Hemisphere Publications, 1974.
10. McLean P: Behavior therapy. Presented at the Society of Psychotherapy Research Panel on Outcome Studies of Depression. Boston, June 12, 1975.
11. Rush A: Cognitive therapy vs. pharmacotherapy. Presented at the Society of Psychotherapy Research Panel on Outcome Studies of Depression. Boston, June 12, 1975.
12. Shaw B: Cognitive therapy vs. behavior therapy. Presented at the Society of Psychotherapy Research Panel on Outcome Studies of Depression. Boston, June 12, 1975.

14

Planning a Total Treatment Program for the Hospitalized Depressed Patient

ROBERT W. GIBSON

It has been estimated that each year some 20 million persons in the United States suffer from depression. In 1971 there were 275,555 admissions for depression to inpatient psychiatric facilities accounting for 22.5% of the total admissions. At 135.3 admissions per 100,000 population, depression was second only to schizophrenia as a cause for psychiatric hospitalization. More than twice as many patients were admitted to outpatient facilities; it is difficult to determine how many were treated by private practitioners and one can only guess how many millions suffering from depression went untreated.

As has been pointed out in this book, the term *depression* has been used loosely to describe the normal response to certain stressful situations, the affective state of depression, the constellation of symptoms that make up the depressive syndrome, and what is postulated to be a specific disease entity and sometimes to identify an underlying character structure predisposing the individual to symptoms of depression.

Depression can at times occur as a symptom in virtually all psychiatric disorders but is the predominant characteristic of four diagnostic entities: manic-depressive disorders, both cyclical and depressed type; involutional reactions; psychotic depressive reactions; and neurotic depressive reactions.

Although classification has been discussed in detail in the first chapter of this book, I should like to summarize the distinguishing characteristics of the categories of the current DSMII classification. Patients suffering from manic-depressive reactions have recurrent attacks charac-

ROBERT W. GIBSON • Sheppard and Enoch Pratt Hospital, Towson, Maryland.

terized by disturbances in affect ranging from elation to depression, by alterations in psychomotor activity from hyperactivity to underactivity, and by disturbances in the thought processes from flight of ideas to marked retardation.

Involutionally depressed patients show most of the clinical characteristics of acute depression, but instead of displaying psychomotor retardation they most commonly are apprehensive and anxious.

Patients with psychotic depressive reactions develop symptoms promptly in response to a clear-cut precipitating event. They are severely depressed and commonly misinterpret reality, occasionally to the point of being delusional. Inasmuch as the distinction between the psychotic and the neurotic depressive reaction is as much quantitative as qualitative, there is some question as to whether it is a valid diagnostic entity.

Patients having neurotic depressive disorders show a variable clinical picture. Symptoms are more responsive to external stimuli and as a consequence rather changeable. Anxiety and other neurotic symptoms are frequently present. Feelings of guilt, hopelessness, and worthlessness may occur but not to the extreme seen in the psychotic depressions. The neurotic patient shows more subjective evidence of depression than objective signs.

Severe depressive symptoms often occur in response to somatic disease in such a way that they override the manifestations of the primary process. Such depressions are common in hypertensive cardiovascular disease, uremia, intracranial lesions, cerebral arteriosclerosis, infectious diseases, toxic deliriums, and drug withdrawal states.

Data from our experience at Sheppard Pratt give some indication of the clinical problems encountered in the various depressive disorders. Approximately 32% of patients admitted are diagnosed as suffering from one of the major categories of depression. This is somewhat higher than the previously quoted 1971 national figure of 22.5% but, in general, private psychiatric hospitals admit a higher percentage of patients suffering from depression. Seven percent of the patients admitted to Sheppard Pratt suffer from depressions of psychotic proportions including involutional reactions, manic-depressive disease, and psychotic depressions. About 25% of the patients have a depressive reaction that is classified *neurotic*.

During the past two years, of those patients with depressions classified as *psychotic* (manic-depressive, involutional, psychotic depression) the age ranged from 20 to 85 with a mean of 57.9; very few of these patients were under the age of 24; the bulk of the patients were equally divided between the 25- to 64-year range and those over 65 years of age. The most common symptoms for both age groups in approximate order of frequency were depression, social withdrawal, sleep disorders, loss of interest, loss of energy, guilt, somatic complaints, and, to a somewhat lesser degree, delusions, confusion, and thought disorders.

Patients having a diagnosis of neurotic depressive reaction ranged in age from 11 to 88 years with a mean age of 36.7. Approximately 30% of these patients were 24 years of age or younger, 55% were in the 25- to 64- year range, and only 15% were over 65. The symptom pattern differed with age. Those under 24 commonly showed depression, hostile aggression, social withdrawal, drug experimentation, running away, guilt, labile affect, self-injury, sleep disorder, loss of interest, sexual problems, and somatic complaints. Those in the 25- to 64-year range complained of depression, marital difficulty, sleep disorder, social withdrawal, guilt, loss of energy, alcohol abuse, somatic complaints, anxiety, self-injury, and loss of interest. Those over 65 characteristically showed depression, somatic complaint, sleep disorder, social withdrawal, and loss of interest.

In all of these groupings, depression itself was the most prominent symptom. All groups showed the constellation of symptoms commonly identified with the depressive syndrome including social withdrawal, loss of interest, sleep disorder, guilt, and loss of energy. Thus, in terms of symptoms, there appears to be a core problem that is present regardless of the diagnosis or age. But in addition there are significant variations depending upon whether the disorder is psychotic or neurotic in character as well as upon the age of the patient. And, of course, individual patients may have significant differences from the common patterns that have been described.

Emergency treatment and crisis intervention are frequently directed just to the symptomatic manifestations of depression without consistent effort at follow-up. Many patients willingly accept such limited treatment because of their wish to deny the severity of symptoms and underlying problems. Treatment programs in hospitals, especially those oriented toward providing intermediate to long-term care, usually attempt to carry treatment beyond just the alleviation of symptoms—hence in the title of this chapter the emphasis on the *total* treatment program.

ETIOLOGY

Inasmuch as a total or comprehensive treatment program implies that an effort will be made to treat not just symptoms, let us briefly review the major theories of etiology. Arising out of various schools of thought, many models have been proposed[1] as an explanation of depression. Psychoanalytic theories include the concepts of aggression turned inward, object loss, loss of self-esteem, and negative cognitive set. Behavioral theories include learned helplessness and loss of reinforcement. Sociologic explanations include loss of role status. Existentialism includes loss of meaning of existence. Biologic theories have proposed disturbances in the metabolism of biogenic amines and neurophysiologic derangement of diencephalic mechanisms.

Psychologic processes appear of particular importance in understanding the milder forms of depressive disorders. In varying degrees most theories identify four factors that may be productive of a depressive disorder: (1) a response to an environmental loss, disappointment, or deprivation leading to affective change; (2) changes in self-esteem arising out of feelings of helplessness, being unloved, and unworthiness; (3) conflicts over aggressive impulses; (4) a preexisting personality structure characterized by narcissism, dependency, and ambivalent object relations.

An attempt has been made to integrate these seemingly diverse explanations by proposing that depressive illness is a psychobiological final common pathway depending on the interaction of several factors: genetic vulnerability, developmental events, psychosocial events, physiological stresses, and personality traits.

It seems premature to conclude that any one of the specific theories of etiology is the only correct one or the most useful in organizing a treatment program. In my own clinical experience with depressed patients I have found virtually all of these concepts useful. The clinical information from different patients may seem to fit various theoretical models. Treatment must be directed toward both presenting symptoms and underlying causes and should include all the therapeutic resources of the hospital.

INDICATIONS FOR HOSPITALIZATION

The psychiatric hospital is designed and organized to provide (1) diagnostic examination, (2) protection of the patient from himself and of society from the patient, (3) interruption of deleterious psychosocial interactions, (4) consistent application of a designed and controlled treatment program, (5) utilization of a prescribed milieu for the patient's treatment. The need for any or all of these may be considered as positive indications for hospital care.

Some specific indications for hospitalization of the depressed patient are continued weight loss, persistent insomnia with early-morning awakening, extreme anxiety, agitation with emotional outbursts, and a continued feeling of hopelessness. Additional indications related to the patient's life situation are intense and disturbing interactions with family or close associates and strained relationships suggesting that some sort of crisis or explosion may occur. Finally, a decision to undertake outpatient treatment should not be made unless the physician feels that some responsive contact has developed between him and the patient in the course of evaluation or prior treatment.

In this chapter I will try to highlight some of the special considerations involved in the treatment of the depressed patient. Coordination of the treatment program is essential because the therapeutic efforts of psychiatrist, social workers, nursing personnel, activity therapists, and others are closely interrelated. For purposes of presentation I will discuss psychotherapy, social service, nursing care and activity therapy, drug therapy, and electrotherapy separately, but the effectiveness of each depends upon close communication and integration in a team effort.

TREATMENT PROGRAM

Psychotherapy

During the psychotic phase the aim of treatment for most depressed patients should be to provide support and protection. Attempts to uncover unconscious material at this time may intensify the patient's anxiety and even increase the likelihood of suicide. Establishing and maintaining a therapeutic relationship can be extremely difficult. The therapist must be flexible in approach; for example, it may be helpful to vary the length of interviews in accordance with the clinical state of the patient—relatively brief, frequent interviews are often preferable for the underactive, retarded patient.

In accordance with the patient's needs, the therapist must actively seek to establish communication in whatever manner seems to work whether it be support, challenge, reassurance, scolding, uncritical acceptance, or annoyance. It is helpful if the patient comes to see the physician as a friendly and powerful figure capable of providing support and gratifying dependency needs. Common sense alterations in the patient's life patterns through environmental manipulation should be undertaken as appropriate. The therapist should be willing to allow the patient to use him as a temporary replacement for object loss.

Implicit in this approach is a commitment to continue treatment, possibly of a long-term nature. The major part of therapeutic work ordinarily must be carried out during the remission of the psychotic episode. Laying the groundwork by establishing a positive alliance during the psychotic period is likely to be the factor determining whether the patient will continue in more active treatment.

In the case of the neurotically depressed patient a supportive approach at the outset is also generally indicated. Because such a patient is likely to be more verbal than the psychotic patient, ventilation is often effective. Even though uncovering techniques and interpretation are best deferred until some relief from the acute symptoms has been achieved, it is often possible to help the patient to delineate and clarify the problem areas. Achieving a consensus concerning the problem areas may provide the therapist with the leverage needed to persuade the patient to continue insight psychotherapy. This is not to suggest that in all cases such therapy is indicated or necessary. Depression occurring in response to severe crisis situations may be resolved promptly with little need for continued care. The problem is that many depressed patients utilize massive denial as a defense against serious conflicts and underlying personality disorders. For such patients continued psychotherapy in accordance with usual therapeutic principles is essential following the resolution of the acute symptoms, be they of psychotic or neurotic proportions.

In the initial phase of treatment individual psychotherapy rather than group therapy is indicated. The severely depressed patient is likely to be disruptive to a group and derive little support from the experience. During later phases, group therapy, sometimes in combination with individual therapy, can be beneficial.

Social Service

As with all hospitalized patients the family members are profoundly affected by the patient's hospitalization. Failure on their part to understand the nature of the problem may compound the difficulties for the patient, and conversely family members can become an important resource in the patient's treatment if they can become involved and assisted through social casework.

For the depressed patient, particularly the neurotically depressed patient, family members may give considerable insight into the nature of the stresses to which the patient was exposed. In many instances, the actual relationships within the family may be a major source of conflict. Social casework is obviously indicated in such situations.

Family therapy is often of value, particularly with younger patients. A series of four to six weekly family therapy sessions, including the patient, significant family members, the social worker, and the primary therapist can assist in understanding the psychodynamics of the patient's illness, can facilitate the patient's therapy, and enhance social casework with the family.

Nursing Care and Activity Therapy

The depressed patient must be protected against the ever-present danger of suicide. This requires reasonably close and frequent observation. Obvious hazards should be minimized but not to the point of creating an oppressive, dehumanizing atmosphere. In years past the attempt was sometimes made to create an environment in which it was physically impossible for the patient to commit suicide. This simply does not work; the depressed patient determined to commit suicide can do so despite the most relentless system of precautions. A rigorous regimen, emphasizing restriction and control, can actually increase the risk of suicide and in addition interfere with activities and experiences that may be therapeutic.

The reasons for staff concern and the purpose of the limits imposed should be clearly and candidly explained to the patient. Although staff members cannot shift their responsibility, the patient group is sometimes more attuned and better able to help their fellow patients. Open discussion at patient–staff meetings can assist other patients to see that self-destructive behavior is as much a matter of group concern as any other symptom.

Other symptoms of the depressed patient requiring attention, especially in psychotic patients, are serious weight loss, dehydration, sleep disturbance, and neglect of personal hygiene. If unattended, these symptoms can become problems in their own right. It is particularly important that staff deal with these symptoms in a manner that conveys concern, offers some gratification of dependency needs, and conveys the message that tangible measures are available to help the patient.

Special care must be exercised in the use of sedatives because of the tendency of depressed patients to become overly dependent or even addicted. It may be best to withhold sedation even though this means that a patient gets only a few hours sleep for several nights. In my experience, sedatives in the long run are not of a great deal of help. After several weeks of regular use of sedatives, the patient is likely to be dependent on the medication, tired most of the day, and still not sleeping. It may be far better for night staff to spend time with the patient who complains of trouble sleeping rather than to automatically give PRN sedatives.

The patient's daily program should be planned to keep him active. This usually requires considerable effort on the part of the staff to overcome retardation and the tendency to withdraw. If by discovering the patient's interest one can motivate him to engage in activities, it is ideal. Much of the time a consistent push from staff is required. It is impossible to generalize about the best approach but staff must at a minimum convey an expectation that the patient will participate in hospital activities and over time expect a gradual expansion in participation.

To the degree possible, the program of activities should be individualized to meet each patient's needs. Physical activity on a level appropriate to the patient's condition is useful in overcoming many of the secondary symptoms of depression. Participation in activities that bring personal contact with staff and other patients is helpful in overcoming object loss. Activity therapies that offer an opportunity for expression of affect—for example, art therapy and dance therapy—are particularly valuable to many patients.

Therapeutic work programs are helpful in enhancing self-esteem. Sometimes it is feasible for the patient to continue some work related to his occupation. Such a decision should be weighed quite carefully. Maintaining these ties may be helpful to the patient's self-esteem, may overcome some of the sense of hopelessness, and facilitate return to productive activities. If the motivation for continued work stems mostly from guilt, a wish to deny the existence of problems, or an effort to avoid involvement in the hospital program, then the continuance of prehospital work activities may be antitherapeutic.

Obviously, the range of possibilities for an individual activity schedule is great. It is essential that a careful diagnostic evaluation be carried out by an experienced activity therapist in consultation with the primary therapist and other members of the treatment team. This makes it possible to incorporate the plan for activity therapy into an overall individualized treatment plan.

The attitudes and reactions of staff members are absolutely critical in the treatment of the depressed patient. Feelings of depression and indeed some of the secondary symptoms are a part of the life experience of every person. This may make it easier for the staff to appreciate the nature of the patient's experiences and to develop an empathic relationship. This very advantage may create a problem inasmuch as the patient's symptoms may seem similar to experiences that staff members have had. Staff may thus underestimate the severity of the disorder and enter into collusion with the patient to deny the need for treatment. Some staff members may even take a judgmental, moralistic approach, exhorting the patient simply to shape up and stop indulging himself.

Depressed patients frequently seek help in a clinging, manipulative fashion. While ostensibly presenting themselves as helpless and at the mercy of the staff, they may actually be quite demanding and controlling. For example, it is often terribly difficult to end an interview with depressed patients as they convey that their needs have not been met and that separation may be shattering. Although pleading for help, depressed patients often seem determined to prove that absolutely nothing can be done to help—they are intent on proving that their situation is completely hopeless.

In trying to help the depressed patient, staff members frequently overextend themselves. When the patient does not respond, it engenders a feeling of hopelessness. The staff member is denied any gratification from his therapeutic efforts and feels angry. But such feelings seem quite improper since the patient seems so pitiful that it is not right to direct rage toward him. This can lead to a pattern of mechanistic response or avoidance of the patient. For example, rather than listen to the patient's expression of hopelessness it is easier to shift attention to a secondary symptom that can be dealt with by offering medication.

Whether object loss is considered to be the cause of depression, it does seem that virtually all depressed patients feel that there is an actual or potential loss of meaningful relationships. Thus it is essential that staff members maintain contact and seek to increase involvement with the depressed patient. This means carefully guarding against a pattern of avoidance. If such begins to develop, then efforts should be made to identify the reasons so that active steps can be taken to overcome it. It follows from what has been said previously that a common problem on the part of staff is the difficulty involved in the patient's clinging, demanding behavior while he simultaneously frustrates all efforts to provide assistance. Open discussion and confrontation of the patient around this issue may sometimes be necessary.

Drug Therapy

The use of chemical agents has an important place in the treatment of patients suffering from depression. Generally speaking the tricyclic antidepressants (especially imipramine and amitryptiline) are considered to be the drugs of choice. MAO inhibitors are generally reserved for patients who have not responded to the trial of the tricyclic drugs. They must be used with considerable caution because of the possibility of serious side effects.

Lithium has been found to be especially helpful in the treatment of the manic-depressive patient. There is strong evidence for a prophylactic action of lithium in recurrent affective disorders, both of the bipolar and of the unipolar type. The data do not, however, provide reliable quantitative measures of the efficacy of the treatment. There is suggestive evidence that the long-term administration of tricyclic antidepressant drugs may have a prophylactic action against recurrence of depression, but in bipolar depressions lithium seems superior for prophylaxis.[2]

It is beyond the scope of this chapter to consider in detail the indications for various drugs, the dosage schedules, and handling of side reactions. These issues have been addressed in the chapters by Kline and Cole. My comments are limited to some general principles. Unless there is some extenuating circumstance such as sharp limitation on the length of hospital stay or severe and dangerous symptoms, the initiation of antidepressants should be deferred for at least several days. Admission to a psychiatric hospital and the related consequences can have a profound effect on the patient's symptoms. If medication is initiated immediately, it is difficult to differentiate between what may be an effect of the medication and what may have resulted from such factors as removal from a stressful situation, gratification of the patient's dependency needs, and the establishment of a therapeutic relationship in which the patient may, for the first time, be able to share his feelings.

Several years ago I served as principal investigator in an NIMH collaborative research study on depression in which a continuation of serious depressive symptoms to the third day of hospitalization was required for inclusion of a patient in the project. It was quite illuminating and more than a bit frustrating to find how many patients, severely depressed on admission, responded so rapidly to the hospital milieu that by the third day they were almost completely asymptomatic and had to be excluded from the study. The point is that utilization of medication within a hospital setting provides an opportunity to assess whether the psychopharmacologic action of the drug is of significance. It permits the trial and error needed to determine what dosage level is required for a therapeutic effect. The patient's tolerance of higher dosages can be checked because the hospital setting permits close observation for side reactions and protection against their consequences.

Thus I would recommend that if possible the use of medications be deferred until one has established a baseline of the severity of the patient's symptoms and has ascertained that something more than psychotherapy and the organized hospital program is needed. Once initiated the medication should be increased at a reasonably rapid schedule up to usual recommended therapeutic doses (250 to 300 mg daily for most tricyclics) so long as serious side reactions do not occur. The medication should then be continued for a minimum of three to four weeks and longer if symptoms persist. This approach will provide the patient with the benefits to be derived from drug treatment while simultaneously permitting an assessment of the effectiveness, required dosage, and incidence of side reactions.

Electrotherapy

Electrotherapy has been widely used as a specific treatment for depression. Some advocate that it should be administered promptly, even on an outpatient basis to treat or abort depressive attacks.

I must acknowledge some bias against this approach, even though it may have some pragmatic value. In my view, depression arises out of the stresses on the person as balanced against both psychological and physical vulnerability. Ideally I would like to help the patient to find better ways of coping with the stresses and if possible open a way toward psychological change that will diminish his vulnerability and consequently the likelihood of further attacks. Initiating electrotherapy immediately would seem to preclude both these possibilities.

As a consequence I would reserve electrotherapy for those patients who have not responded to a reasonable trial of hospital treatment including an adequate trial of antidepressant medication. Ordinarily it would be limited to depressions of psychotic proportion and particularly the involutional depressions. Admittedly, an exception should be made in instances where electroshock may be administered as a lifesaving measure where the self-destructive behavior of the patient is intense. (For a similar view of electroconvulsive therapy, the reader is referred to Chapter 6 by Kline.)

Discharge

As already indicated, continued treatment of the depressed patient after discharge from the hospital is of particular importance. Ideally, there should be continuity of care through a single process that includes various levels of support by hospitalization, day treatment, outpatient care, and so forth.

The move out of the hospital is a decisive step. After discharge the patient will again be subjected to a variety of stresses, sometimes more intense because of his hospitalization. Inevitably, there will be certain parts of the treatment program that must be discontinued. On many occasions I have seen a sudden recurrence of acute and severe symptoms in patients who appeared by every standard to have made a good recovery during hospitalization and had developed a reasonable life plan for the postdischarge period.

Of particular significance is the activation of separation anxiety as the patient perceives the discharge to be a loss of a dependency relationship. To combat this tendency every effort should be made to arrange the discharge as a series of graded steps. While still in the hospital, the patient may be able to reestablish significant ties to family, friends, and work. If a change in primary therapist is necessary, the relationship should be established prior to the patient's discharge. The goal is to develop a plan so that the patient at the time of discharge is moving toward tangible, already established relationships rather than simply losing what he has found to be so valuable during his hospital experience.

Adolescents and the Elderly

Although the general principles of treatment described apply to all age ranges, a specific comment about adolescents and the elderly seems in order. The incidence of depression in the elderly is particularly high.

Over 40% of the patients over age 65 admitted to Sheppard Pratt fall into the major diagnostic classification of depression. Even this does not tell the whole story: 70 to 80% of the older patients have depression as a major symptom.

The high incidence of depression in the elderly is not surprising. The life situation of the older person is likely to lead to a serious object loss. Of our admissions to Sheppard Pratt, we find that 70 to 80% of these patients have sustained some obvious loss just prior to hospitalization such as death of a relative or friend, failing health or loss of functional capacity, and changes in living pattern such as retirement.

Social casework is especially important with older patients. Changes in their environmental situations are often precipitating causes of the depression and their correction may be crucial to successful treatment.

Quite frequently the psychological stresses related to the depression cause symptoms suggestive of an organic disturbance. Such symptoms frequently clear with the correction of physical problems and the removal from psychological stress. It is disturbing to speculate how many patients may have been denied appropriate treatment because they were written off as hopelessly brain-damaged.

Unfortunately, many clinicians have little interest in working with older patients. They see them as unsuitable for any form of psychotherapy. They are unjustifiably pessimistic about their prognosis. In evaluating the treatment outcome of these older depressed patients at Sheppard Pratt, it was somewhat surprising and most gratifying to find that over 90% recovered sufficiently that they could return to the prehospital level of functioning.

We have found the incidence of depressive neuroses to be substantially higher in adolescents than previously suspected; depressive reactions are diagnosed in about one-third of our patients under the age of 17. There is some indication that the frequency of suicidal attempts is increasing in younger patients. And beyond that, much of the adolescents' behavior is self-destructive, as for example when they expose themselves to seriously hazardous situations. The depressive quality of the disorder is frequently obscured in the adolescent by hostile aggressive behavior, running away, drug experimentation, hyperactivity, and promiscuous sexual activity. Hospitalization limits and controls such behavior with the result that the depressive symptomatology often becomes manifest. This is generally a favorable sign.

Antidepressants must be used with considerable caution in the younger patients because of their proclivity for misusing such drugs in efforts to achieve some kind of high. We have found that major tranquilizers such as thioridazine that also relieve depression are sometimes superior to antidepressants because of their therapeutic action not only for the depression but also for agitation, hyperactivity, and aggressiveness. In my experience, the treatment results of depressions in the adolescent and in elderly patients tend to be favorable.

Conclusion

Depression is a health problem of major proportions. Hospitalization at some stage of treatment is indicated for a substantial number of patients; an optimal treatment will for most patients include a period of outpatient care as well. Treatment efforts should be directed toward increasing the capacity for the person suffering from depression to cope and attempting to modify the impact of various stresses. Until further research has fully demonstrated the various causes, an open-minded approach is indicated for the treatment of depression. Psychotherapy, environmental manipulation, and drugs should all be a part of a coordinated treatment effort. Fortunately, a carefully planned total treatment program is rewarded by favorable outcomes in a high percentage of patients.

REFERENCES

1. Akiskal HS, McKinney WT: An overview of recent research in depression. *Arch. Gen. Psychiatry 32:*285–305, 1975.
2. Prien R, Klett CJ, Caffey E: Lithium carbonate and imipramine in the prevention of affective episodes. *Arch. Gen. Psychiatry 29:*40–225, 1973.

Index